Erectile Dysfunction and Vascular Disease

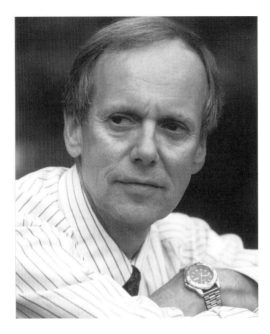

Dr Mike Kirby

Erectile Dysfunction and Vascular Disease

Dr Michael Kirby FRCP

Director of HertNet—The Hertfordshire
Primary Care Research Network
The Surgery
Nevells Road
Letchworth
Herts
UK

Blackwell
Publishing

© 2003 by Blackwell Publishing Ltd
Blackwell Publishing, Inc., 350 Main Street, Malden, Massachusetts 02148-5018, USA
Blackwell Publishing Ltd, Osney Mead, Oxford OX2 0EL, UK
Blackwell Publishing Asia Pty Ltd, 550 Swanston Street, Carlton South, Victoria 3053, Australia
Blackwell Verlag GmbH, Kurfürstendamm 57, 10707 Berlin, Germany

First published 2003 by Blackwell Publishing Ltd

Library of Congress Cataloging-in-Publication Data
Kirby, Michael, FRCP
    Erectile dysfunction and vascular disease / Mike Kirby.
        p. ; cm.
    Includes bibliographical references and index.
    ISBN 1-4051-0753-7
    1. Impotence.   I. Title.
    [DNLM: 1. Impotence, Vasculogenic. 2. Impotence.
WJ 709 K58e 2003]
    RC889.K535 2003
    616.6'92 -- dc21

2002014091

ISBN 1-4051-0753-7

A catalogue record for this title is available from the British Library

Set in 9/12pt Photina by Sparks Computer Solutions, Oxford, UK
Printed and bound in Great Britain at Ashford Colour Press, Gosport

Commissioning Editor: Stuart Taylor
Managing Editor: Heather Johnston
Production Editor: Nick Morgan
Production Controller: Chris Downs

For further information on Blackwell Publishing, visit our website:
http://www.blackwellpublishing.com

Contents

Forewords, vi

Preface, ix

CHAPTER 1: Erectile Dysfunction—an introduction, 1

CHAPTER 2: Government Initiatives in Men's Health, 24

CHAPTER 3: Identification and Management of Risk Factors, 32

CHAPTER 4: Guiding the Patient, 49

CHAPTER 5: Cardiovascular Disease and Sex, 64

CHAPTER 6: Well Man and Erectile Dysfunction Clinics in General Practice, 85

CHAPTER 7: Nurses in the Front Line, 102

CHAPTER 8: Case Studies, 108

CHAPTER 9: Most Frequently Asked Questions, 115

Index, 121

Forewords

As a diabetologist with an interest in the management of erectile dysfunction (ED), I am only too aware of how neglected this condition has been. This was perhaps acceptable in the days when ED was thought to be due to witchcraft and/or the wrath of God, and in any case there was no effective treatment. Now that ED is recognised as an organic problem related to significant underlying disease, and over 80% of men can be successfully treated, surely to ignore ED is negligent. It is quite unacceptable to ignore any other organ failure, so why the penis?

The reason for potential neglect must surely be that sexual function and activity remain, at least for heterosexual men, a taboo subject—men and their professional health carers are embarrassed. Male health, including male sexual health, is supposed to be a healthcare priority, yet official guidance seldom mentions ED. The focus tends to be on transmissible sexual diseases and high-risk sexual practice. Disease and diabetes detection and early management are a greater priority of the national (health) service frameworks. Yet, once again the value of treating ED in this context has been underestimated to date. The prescribing regulations for ED treatment can discourage men from approaching a healthcare professional with their health problems, men in whom ED may well be the first sign of serious underlying disease. Encouraging men to present with their ED could be used as an opportunity for screening and early diagnosis of these important conditions.

This book is a very useful addition to the increasing educational material available on the topic of ED. It is refreshingly different to many other books on the topic. It concentrates on the relationship between vascular diseases and ED, and particularly coronary artery disease. Many myths still abound regarding 'sex and the heart' and this should help dispel many of them. The book also emphasizes more general aspects of the problem of men's health, both general and sexual, and the psychology involved. It also has useful chapters discussing political aspects, general aspects of ED management and service delivery. Such material should help to encourage more nurses and doctors in both primary and secondary care to overcome their inhibitions and take a more active role in the management of ED. Have a read!

Bill Alexander
Consultant Physician (Diabetes)

Sex is an important part of life and it is everyone's right to enjoy a sexual relationship. When an organic disorder interferes with an individual's ability to enjoy sex, it is our responsibility as healthcare professionals to help restore the sexual relationship. We are unfortunately not very good at fulfilling our responsibilities, mainly due to lack of awareness of the problem. When this is combined with lack of education on how to manage sexual dysfunction and patients' reluctance to volunteer the problem in the first place, we have a significant unmet need which causes unnecessary distress.

Mike Kirby's book addresses these issues in a practical way and should help us overcome the barriers to discussion and advice. The book is ideally suited to family practice but will also be of value to hospital-based clinics, where ED also needs to be addressed. Given that 70% of patients with ED have vascular disease as the main cause, appropriate emphasis on diabetes and cardiac disease is provided. The management of sexual dysfunction should be a partnership.

The medical partners (hospital, primary care) need to combine their expertise to help the partners with the problems. ED may be a man's problem but it is a couple's concern and this book goes a long way towards helping us identify, manage and restore a satisfying sexual relationship.

Graham Jackson
Consultant Cardiologist

The nurse's role has changed dramatically over the past couple of years and is continuing to evolve, as nurses take on a more varied and broader remit within the NHS. This is being recognized at government and practice levels. One of the most important advances is maximizing the benefits of nurses acting as the first point of contact. This has undoubtedly influenced NHS policy development. Plans for setting up a supplementary prescribing scheme are progressing rapidly, enabling nurses to prescribe medications for long-term conditions such as diabetes mellitus and hypertension.

Erectile dysfunction, especially given its link to underlying chronic disease, is a key area where nurses can and should be encouraged to become more of an integral part of the healthcare team. Through routine diabetes and cardiovascular clinics, Well Man clinics and general health checks, nurses are in an ideal position to proactively identify and manage ED. Good communication skills are vital if men are to be encouraged to talk about their ED. The chapter 'Guiding the patient' looks at strategies to help the patient and the healthcare professional feel more comfortable about addressing this sometimes embarrassing and difficult topic.

This book provides information for all primary healthcare professionals on the management of ED in the cardiovascular patient, supporting other resources and practical education programmes specifically tailored to nurses. I am sure nurses will be encouraged to see that their valuable role in managing ED is recognized with a specific chapter dedicated to nurses.

Carole McCallum
Practice Nurse

Erectile dysfunction has traditionally been one of those hidden conditions which has been ignored both by patients and by doctors alike. With the progressive increase in life expectancy, and with the increasing quality of health and life in older people, the number of men who suffer from ED is ever increasing. The advent of effective oral therapy and the publicity that surrounded it brought ED into the public domain in a way that it had never been present before, and as a result there are increasing numbers of men seeking treatment.

Traditionally therapy for ED was the domain of hospital specialists but it is increasingly clear that many men are best managed in the community either by primary care physicians or by nurse specialists. Although therapy in the community is clearly desirable, there are a number of issues that have thus far impeded such approaches. One of these issues is education, and in this excellent book Mike Kirby seeks to redress this issue. As a general practitioner with an interest in men's health, he has considerable experience in the issues surrounding the diagnosis and treatment of ED in the community. This book provides an up-to-date guide and state-of-the-art knowledge for physicians and nurses seeking to treat men with erection problems.

Ian Eardley
Consultant Urologist

Preface

The process of normal erectile function is complex. It requires the co-ordination of a number of psychological, hormonal, neurological and vascular factors. Erectile dysfunction (ED) is the inability to achieve or maintain an erection sufficient for sexual activity. The increasing wealth of research surrounding the causes and effects of ED leaves little doubt that ED can be hugely detrimental to a man's self-esteem and overall quality of life. The availability of new and effective therapies has now made it possible for this extremely common medical condition to be increasingly understood and managed in primary care. The aim of this book is to focus on the importance of the vascular system as a primary cause of ED, the inter-relationship with other causes of ED and optimum approaches to treatment for erection problems.

The most common physical causes of ED are conditions that impair arterial flow to the erectile tissues or disrupt the neuronal system, such as atherosclerosis, hypertension or diabetes. ED may often be the first presenting symptom in men with previously undiagnosed chronic conditions such as cardiovascular disease and diabetes. The proactive identification of ED can not only help restore a sexual relationship, but also enable underlying diseases to be diagnosed at an earlier stage, improving treatment outcomes and helping to fulfil government standards for care such as the National Service Frameworks for Coronary Heart Disease and Diabetes.

Despite cardiovascular disease being one of the increasingly recognized causes of ED, healthcare professionals can be overly cautious when it comes to the day-to-day management of ED in the cardiovascular patient. This book intends to dispel common myths associated with vascular disease, sexual intercourse and ED, providing healthcare professionals with the knowledge and confidence to improve the management of patients with ED. One chapter is specifically dedicated to the increasing scope for practice nurse involvement in identifying and managing men with sexual conditions. Further education and training can equip nurses to help address erection problems and subsequent intimacy issues within a relationship.

It is critical when looking to improve the management of any health issue to focus on practicalities. Erection problems and other sexual conditions can be addressed within the wider context of men's health. Based on my own personal experience, practical advice and guidance for establishing and running a Well Man clinic is offered. Such clinics can provide an ideal opportunity for healthcare professionals to broach the sometimes difficult subject of ED. Information from this text, such as the protocol for the Well Man clinic, can be downloaded from the website www.edvasculardisease.com for use in everyday practice.

It is hoped that this book will complement earlier texts relating to general information on, and advances in, the management of ED. It draws on new evidence and experience for managing ED and highlights the importance of its intrinsic link with vascular disease, an established government healthcare priority.

Mike Kirby

CHAPTER 1

Erectile Dysfunction — an introduction

INTRODUCTION

The term impotence (the term traditionally applied to erection difficulties) derives from the Latin meaning 'loss of power'. This association with a lack of strength and vigour automatically connects the condition with the opposite of all that we consider masculine. For centuries, men have linked their self-respect to the performance of their penis. Therefore, when their penis fails them, they no longer feel like 'real' men [1]. As this physical event affects most men to some degree at some point in their life, the word used to describe the condition should not suggest a sweeping diminution in a man's overall strength and capabilities, as the word 'impotence' does. With this in mind, the term 'erectile dysfunction' (ED) was coined.

ED is defined as the inability to achieve or maintain an erection sufficient for sexual activity and can be either organic or inorganic (i.e. psychological) in origin. As little as 30 years ago it was still believed that the majority of ED cases were inorganic in nature, although by the 1970s and 1980s many experts were starting to believe that ED was increasingly due to organic disease. Today it is broadly accepted that there is rarely a clear-cut cause of ED and that erectile failure is usually due to a complex interaction between a number of psychological and physical factors.

SIZE OF THE PROBLEM

Given that men are notoriously reticent in seeking advice or help with their ED, it is difficult to obtain precise figures on the prevalence of ED in the male population.

It has been suggested that up to 52% of men between the ages of 40 and 70 years will have experienced some degree of ED [2,3]. ED also appears to be age related, with a prevalence of 39% among men 40 years old, and 67% among those 70 years old [2]. As the ageing population is ever-growing, the number of men with ED is set to increase quite startlingly. Based on new estimates of the worldwide prevalence of ED, the present worldwide prevalence of >150 million men with ED is likely to double in the next 25 years, exceeding 300 million men by 2025 [4].

ANATOMY OF THE PENIS

In order to understand fully the physiology of the condition and its underlying causes, it is important first to review the basic structure of the penis (Fig. 1.1).

The penis is a vascular organ which is essentially divided into three cylindrical columns—two corpora cavernosa and the corpus spongiosum. The paired corpora cavernosa, which constitute the bulk of the penis, are surrounded by a thick, non-expansile fibrous sheath (tunica albuginea), which supports the rigidity of erectile function. In the midline, the tunica of the two corpora are fused to form a midline septum. The corpus spongiosum surrounds the urethra and expands distally to form the glans, within which the two corpora cavernosa terminate. The ligament which 'suspends' the erect penis into a position perpendicular to the body when a man is standing, arises from the pubic symphysis and attaches to the deep fascia on the dorsum of the penis.

The three cylinders are enclosed by a sturdy fascial layer (called Buck's fascia), subcutaneous tissue and skin. The cylinders themselves are composed of spongy tissue called trabecular tissue which contain smooth muscle, collagen, elastin, blood vessels and nerves. Within the trabecular tissue are many interconnecting cavities called cavernous spaces. These spaces are lined with vascular endothelium.

Blood supply of the penis

The endothelium lining the cavernous spaces in the corpora cavernosa is supplied with blood via the coiled helicine branches of the cavernosal arteries. These arteries control the flow of blood into the cavernosal spaces and are hence the main resistance vessels of the penis. The bulbar artery supplies the bulb, the corpus spongiosum and the glans. All these arteries are branches of the penile artery, which itself originates from the internal pudendal artery.

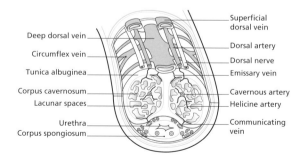

Fig. 1.1 Cross-section of penis showing the blood and nerve supply.

Venous blood drains from the cavernous spaces of the corpus cavernosa through emissary veins which run under the tunica albuginea. These then exit through the tunica albuginea and ultimately drain into the deep dorsal vein and the peri-prostatic venous complex.

Nerve supply of the penis (Fig. 1.2)

The mechanism of erection is largely controlled by the autonomic nervous system, but both the central and the peripheral nervous system play a role. A number of neural pathways to and from the brain influence and sometimes initiate an erectile response. Audiovisual stimuli or sexual fantasy send signals from the brain to the spinal erection centre activating the erectile process, although these pathways can also inhibit the same process, resulting in psychogenic ED. Nerves from the sacral spinal cord (S2–4) are the principal mediators of erection. They receive messages from the central nervous system as well as sensory information from the penis. This initiates a reflex arc that can cause or maintain an erection. Sympathetic nerves from the thoracolumbar cord (T11–L2) control ejaculation and detumescence. Sensory information is contained within the peripheral nerves, which are also responsible for erectile function, particularly maintenance of erection. Ultimate control of erectile function is through the central nervous system, and it is believed that the median preoptic area of the hypothalamus plays an integral part of psychogenic erectile stimulation.

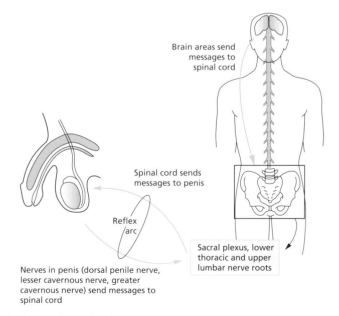

Brain areas send messages to spinal cord

Spinal cord sends messages to penis

Reflex arc

Nerves in penis (dorsal penile nerve, lesser cavernous nerve, greater cavernous nerve) send messages to spinal cord

Sacral plexus, lower thoracic and upper lumbar nerve roots

Fig. 1.2 Nerve pathways involved in erection.

TYPES OF ERECTION
There are three main types of erection in man: 'reflexogenic', 'psychogenic' and 'nocturnal'.

Reflexogenic erections
Direct stimulation of the penis and surrounding tissues can result in an erection. This is probably a reflex response, functioning independently of the brain and higher centres, although under certain circumstances it can be regulated by impulses from above. Erotic thoughts can also facilitate this reflex. A reflex arc is activated from the sacral roots at S2 to S4.

Psychogenic erections
Common in younger men, but decreasing in frequency with increasing age, psychogenic erections are generated primarily through visual, olfactory or imaginative stimuli, and can occur without any direct stimulation to the penis or surrounding tissues. Both the parasympathetic and sympathetic neural pathways are thought to be involved, with sexual input being relayed to the spinal cord at T11 to L2. Visual or imaginative erotic stimuli can improve the response to manual stimuli and vice versa.

Nocturnal and early morning erections (nocturnal penile tumescence)
All men without erectile problems experience on average between four and six erections a night (about 100 min in total duration), of which most are associated with rapid eye movement (REM) sleep. It is thought that the purpose of this is to provide increased oxygen to penile tissues.

If a man presenting with ED has nocturnal erections, it is generally thought that this is indicative of a psychogenic cause of the ED. However, occasionally this may not be the case if the pathways between psychogenic and nocturnal erections are different. Depressed men rarely experience REM sleep and therefore do not have nocturnal or early morning erections. Most waking erections are a result of the psychogenic and reflexogenic pathways working together.

MECHANISM OF ERECTION
Although an erection is largely a vascular event, the activity or tone of the smooth muscle is crucial in controlling the erect or flaccid state of the penis. The two most fundamental events during an erection, arteriolar dilatation and trabecular smooth muscle relaxation, are both determined by the tone of the smooth muscle within them.

Flaccid state
In the flaccid state, the sympathetic nervous system activity maintains constriction of the arterioles and tonic contraction of the cavernosal smooth mus-

cle. Therefore, blood flow through the cavernosal artery into the cavernous spaces remains low, but provides oxygen and other important nutrients.

Erection

In response to sexual stimuli, with or without tactile stimulation of the penis, the parasympathetic nervous system causes dilatation of the cavernosal and coiled helinous arteries and relaxation of the trabecular smooth muscle. This increases the flow of blood into the penis, filling the sinusoidal spaces and causing the penis to engorge with blood. Eventually, such tumescence is reached that the expanding sinusoids compress the venous channels between the tunica albuginea and the peripheral sinusoids. This process reduces and ultimately stops the venous outflow through the emissary veins (veno-occlusive mechanism) and the erection is maintained. Inflow of blood to the corpora cavernosa is minimal at this point. Rigidity can be enhanced through contraction of the perineal muscles.

Detumescence

Detumescence is the reverse of these events, usually after the removal of erotic stimuli or after ejaculation. The resulting increased sympathetic activity increases the tone of the helicine arteries and stimulates contraction of the trabecular smooth muscle. This allows venous outflow from the corpora cavernosa and the corpus spongiosum through decompression of the venous channels. As both orgasm and ejaculation are also mediated by the sympathetic nervous system, detumescence occurs naturally after these events.

The role of nitric oxide-cyclic guanosine monophosphate in penile erection

A number of chemical pathways are involved in the erectile response. However, the most important of these is the nitric oxide-induced cyclic guanosine monophosphate (cGMP) pathway. In response to sexual stimuli, cavernosal nerves and endothelial cells release nitric oxide (NO). NO diffuses into the smooth muscle cells of the corpus cavernosa and activates guanylate cyclase, an enzyme which results in increased synthesis of cGMP. cGMP relaxes the corpus cavernosal smooth muscle by decreasing intracellular calcium, leading to an erection. Detumescence occurs when cGMP is broken down by an enzyme called phosphodiesterase (PDE) type 5 (see Fig. 1.4).

PHYSIOLOGY OF ED

Normal erectile function is a complex process, requiring co-ordination of a number of psychological, hormonal, neurological and vascular factors. If one or more of these factors is disrupted, ED may result. Regardless of the precipitating factor or factors, there is usually a psychogenic component involved, especially if the patient has delayed presenting to their physician, as is often the case.

Table 1.1 Differential diagnosis of psychogenic and organic ED [5].

Psychogenic ED	Organic ED
• Sudden onset	• Gradual onset
• Specific situation	• All circumstances
• Normal nocturnal and early morning erections	• Absent nocturnal and early morning erections
• Relationship problems	• Normal libido and ejaculation
• Problems during sexual development	• Normal sexual development

Psychogenic causes of ED

The pathophysiology of ED of wholly psychogenic cause is often unclear, although as an erection relies partly upon messages based on visual, auditory, olfactory or imaginative stimuli being sent from the brain to the spinal cord, it can be seen how psychological dysfunction might inhibit stimuli from the brain, and block normal erection.

Early morning, self-stimulated and spontaneous nocturnal erections are usually preserved in men with purely psychogenic ED and the ED is often inconsistent, occurring only in certain situations. Also, the onset of ED can often be linked to a distinct precipitating event (e.g. death of a spouse, loss of job, a psychologically traumatic episode of sexual failure—see Table 1.1). Performance anxiety is a common form of psychogenic ED—once a male experiences erectile failure, further attempts at sexual contact may produce anxiety, which could further contribute to a lack of response. Young men are more likely to have ED due to a psychological cause, whereas men over 50 are more likely to have a cause that is organic in nature.

Possible causes of psychogenic ED

- Anxiety or stress due to work, personal or finance-related matters
- Psychological trauma or abuse
- Anxiety about sexual performance or sexual identity
- Sexual problems in the partner
- Relationship/intimacy problems
- Depression
- Psychosis
- Misconceptions/lack of sex education

Organic causes of ED

A progressive loss of erectile function with a gradual loss of sustainable erectile rigidity, often combined with the loss of early morning and nocturnal erections, would lead to the assumption that the ED was organic in origin. Vasculogenic problems are the most common cause of organic ED, but regardless of the primary aetiology, it should be borne in mind that a psychological element frequently coexists with the organic cause (Table 1.2).

Causes of organic ED were, until recently, thought to relate primarily to vascular and neuropathic dysfunction, including defective blood flow into the penis, endocrine pathology, an inefficient veno-occlusive mechanism, or peripheral autonomic neuropathy. However, increased attention has recently been paid to the structure and function of the corporal smooth muscle and the role of the endothelium. The most common organic causes of ED are conditions that impair arterial flow to the erectile tissues or disrupt the neuronal circuitry (Fig. 1.3). The physiology behind risk factors and underlying conditions associated with ED are examined in depth in Chapter 4.

OVERVIEW OF TREATMENTS FOR ED
A number of new treatments for ED have become available over the last decade, and as further research into additional treatment options continues to be conducted throughout the world, the range of available treatments will increase. With this ever expanding range it will be vital for physicians in the future to ensure that they are aware of all the evidence for all the available treatments in order to make an informed decision in discussion with the patient/partner on the most effective and appropriate treatment for their individual patients.

PSYCHOSEXUAL THERAPY
Psychosexual therapy aims to take into account all aspects of a patient's life that might have contributed to his sexual and relationship difficulties. Partners are encouraged to attend therapy whenever possible. It is particularly appropriate for those patients for whom performance anxiety is a large part of the problem, and in addition to this it is also important to identify other relationship problems, lack of sexual performance, difficulty with intimacy and major or minor depression. If depression is diagnosed and deemed to be severe enough for medical treatment, caution is advised, as many antidepressant medications can in themselves result in ED, and serotonin re-uptake-inhibiting antidepressants often produce delayed ejaculation. Even if the problem has an organic cause, psychosexual therapy may be a good starting point for treatment, either as a stand-alone treatment or complemented with pharmaceutical treatments, as there may be a psychological component to the condition, especially if the patient has suffered for a number of years.

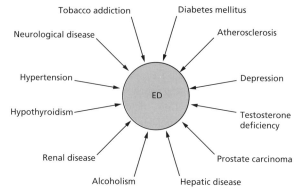

Fig. 1.3 Common organic causes of ED.

ORAL THERAPY
Sildenafil citrate (Viagra™)

Since its launch in 1998, sildenafil has become among the most widely prescribed medications, with nearly 120 million prescriptions written for 20 million men worldwide and has revolutionized the management of ED. It is now the recommended first-line therapy for the majority of ED patients.

Mode of action

Sildenafil was originally researched as an anti-anginal agent because of its vasodilatory effects. However, it was not until the men in the clinical trials began reporting on the unexpected side-effect of enhanced erections that it was realized that an effective oral treatment of ED may have inadvertently been discovered. A subsequent decade and a half of research and development into the effects of sildenafil on ED led to its launch in 1998.

Sildenafil is a selective inhibitor of PDE5, the enzyme responsible for the breakdown of cGMP, which leads to smooth muscle contraction and detumescence. When the NO–cGMP pathway is activated, as occurs with sexual stimulation, inhibition of PDE5 by sildenafil causes increased concentrations of cGMP in the corpus cavernosum, hence prolonging smooth muscle relaxation in erectile function (Fig. 1.4). This explains how sildenafil helps to restore *natural* erectile function in the presence of sexual stimulation [6]. It is not an aphrodisiac and will not have any effect in the absence of sexual stimulation.

Administration

- Recommended dosing regimen for sildenafil is 50 mg taken 30 min to 4 h prior to sexual activity.

Table 1.2 Efficacy of sildenafil in different patient populations.

Patient group	n	Placebo (% patients reporting improvement in erections)	Sildenafil (% patients reporting improvement in erections)	P-value
Hypertension [8]	1218 (sildenafil or placebo)	21	70	<0.0001
Coronary heart disease [10]	213 (sildenafil) 102 (placebo)	20	70	<0.0001
Depression [11]	66 (sildenafil) 75 (placebo)	11	91	<0.0001
Diabetes [12]	131 (sildenafil) 127 (placebo)	10	56	<0.001
Multiple sclerosis [13]	103 (sildenafil) 112 (placebo)	24	89	<0.0001
Spinal injury [14]	143 (sildenafil and placebo)	5	78	<0.001
Radical prostatectomy [15]	87 (sildenafil) 55 (placebo)	15	43	<0.001
TURP [15]	109 (sildenafil) 62 (placebo)	34	61	<0.001

- Treatment with sildenafil should be attempted on at least eight separate occasions, starting at 50 mg and titrating up to 100 mg dose, before considering alternative treatments.
- If sildenafil is taken with or after a high fat meal, the rate of absorption is reduced—the efficacy will not be affected, it will just take longer for the treatment to take effect.
- The maximum recommended dosing frequency for sildenafil is once per day. This is in keeping with the average man's desired frequency of sex.
- Sexual stimulation is necessary.

Side-effects and contraindications

Any side-effects are mild and transient—the most commonly reported being headache, facial flushing and dyspepsia [7]. Less frequently reported side-effects include nasal congestion, and changes in colour vision. These side-effects are usually dose related and completely reversible when the drug is withdrawn. In clinical studies, discontinuation due to adverse events has been proven to be no higher in men taking the active drug than in those receiving placebo.

Sildenafil's haemodynamic profile is similar to a nitrate preparation, causing a modest fall in pulmonary artery pressure and an 8–10 mmHg fall in systolic blood pressure [8]. When sildenafil and nitrates are administered together, clinically significant reductions in blood pressure can occur which may be potentially harmful to the patient. Therefore, sildenafil's concurrent use with nitrates of any form, either episodic or continuous, is contraindicated. Due to the potential for lowering of blood pressure, taking inhaled nitrates such as amyl nitrate (poppers) with sildenafil should also be strongly discouraged. Caution is

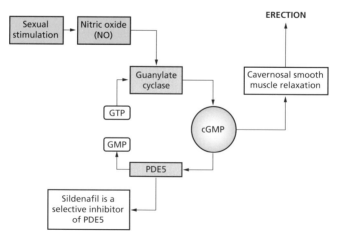

Fig. 1.4 Site of action of sildenafil on the nitric oxide–cGMP mechanism.

advised with NO donors such as nicorandil. If sildenafil is considered the most appropriate treatment for the patient (aside from the nitrates), it is worth considering transferring the patient to an alternative anti-ischaemic therapy (see Chapter 9). This is possible in most angina patients after careful assessment.

Response rates

It should be noted that at the time of writing there are no published head-to-head studies directly comparing pharmacological treatments.

An overall response rate of approximately 80% has been reported when using sildenafil to treat men with ED of various causes [9] (Table 1.2).

Summary of sildenafil

Advantages
- Effective in up to 80% of men
- Non-invasive
- Well tolerated
- Suitable for most men with ED
- Provides a natural response to sexual stimulation

Disadvantages
- Contraindicated in patients taking any form of nitrate therapy
- Systemic side-effects (although generally mild and transient)

Apomorphine (Uprima™)

Apomorphine has long been known as an erectogenic agent in both animals and men. Its use as a subcutaneous agent was first demonstrated more than a decade ago. Unfortunately, direct injection of apomorphine results in severe nausea and vomiting. A sublingual formulation of apomorphine was developed, now known as Uprima, which maintains erectogenic function while decreasing adverse events [16].

Mode of action (Fig. 1.5)

Improving the incoming erectile neural signal will enhance the cellular response within the entire vascular bed serviced by the nerves—within the limits of the unused capacity of the smooth muscle. It therefore follows that improving or increasing the central pro-erectile neural signalling to the spinal centres or manipulating the spinal centres themselves could be a viable treatment of ED. Apomorphine stimulates postsynaptic dopamine receptors (D1 and D2) specifically in the paraventricular and supraoptic nuclei of the hypothalamus, hence acting centrally on the parasympathetic erectile stimulus and leading to erections and yawning in animals.

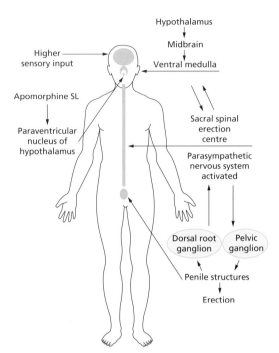

Fig. 1.5 Apomorphine stimulates postsynaptic dopamine receptors (D1 and D2).

Administration

- Recommended dosing regime is to commence patient on 2 mg and adjust up to a maximum of 3 mg as needed [17].
- The drug is taken sublingually and its onset of action is between 15 and 25 min.
- Average median duration of erection is 13 min [17].

Side-effects and contraindications

Because the dopamine receptors stimulate the chemotrigger zone in the brain, treatment can lead to nausea (the most common side-effect, 2–4.8%), hypotension (rarely), and occasional vomiting (0.5%), although these problems tend to be dose related and diminish with repeated exposure to the drug. Other adverse effects include sweating, dizziness and somnolence. The most serious adverse effect (although only a small risk—about 1 in 500) is syncope, although this is nearly always precluded by prodromal events such as nausea, lightheadedness, sweating, and hypotension of vasovagal origin. It is therefore important that the prescribing physician advises caution to the patient if he is trying apomorphine for the first time or is increasing the dose from 2 mg to 3 mg. Nausea, vomiting and glossitis are more common in patients receiving 4 mg than 2 or 3 mg [18,19].

Response rates

- Proportion of attempts resulting in erections firm enough for intercourse found to be 49% with 3 mg dose [19].
- Men with coronary artery disease respond at a rate of 42% [19] of attempts at sexual intercourse being successful, and men with diabetes at 39%.
- Efficacy of Uprima increases with repeat exposure (at least eight doses).
- In patients responding to apomorphine SL, over 90% of attempts are successful over 18 months [20].

Because of the drug's mode of action, apomorphine may be particularly effective in younger men with mild to moderate ED and in patients with spinal injuries. It may also be useful in cases where sildenafil is contraindicated (i.e. if the patient is on nitrates, although caution is still advised) or in those patients whose wish is for a rapid and spontaneous erection (e.g. patients not in a stable relationship). Apomorphine has not yet been evaluated in patients following radical prostatectomy or radiotherapy, but it is not likely to help men who have a complete subsacral nerve lesion, since the parasympathetic stimulus will not be deliverable.

Summary of apomorphine

Advantages
- Effective in 40–50% of men
- Non-invasive
- Restores natural response to sexual stimulation
- Well tolerated
- Can be taken by patients on nitrates

Disadvantages
- Efficacy is not as high as other oral treatments
- As medication must dissolve sublingually, this can interfere with foreplay (kissing, oral stimulation)

NEW ORAL THERAPIES ON THE HORIZON

At the time of writing, tadalafil and vardenafil (phosphodiesterase Type 5 (PDE5) inhibitors—the same drug class as sildenafil) are currently in global Phase III trials. Vardenafil appears to be as effective at treating ED in men with

1

diabetes as with other physical causes of ED. It has also been shown to provide a clear improvement in rigidity and duration of erections as the dose increases [21]. Tadalafil has similar efficacy rates and a duration of 16–24 h [22]. The optimum dose of tadalafil appears to be 20 mg. There are no comparative data yet for the PDE5 inhibitors. Like sildenafil, side-effects for vardenafil and tadalafil appear to be mild and transient, and include headache and dyspepsia. Vardenafil has been associated with minor vision disturbance, while tadalafil has received reports of back pain and myalgia, but has a low incidence of facial flushing and has not been linked to any visual disturbances.

INTRACAVERNOSAL INJECTION THERAPY
Mode of action
Direct intracavernosal injection was first discovered in the early 1980s. The drug currently licensed for use in intracavernosal injection therapy is prostaglandin E_1 (PGE_1—alprostadil or Caverject®).

PGE_1 occurs naturally and is a potent smooth muscle relaxant. It acts on the specific receptors on the surface of the smooth muscle cell, thus stimulating the enzyme adenylate cyclase. This enzyme converts adenosine triphosphate (ATP) to cyclic adenosine monophosphate (cAMP). This rise in cAMP leads to a fall in the intracellular calcium and subsequent smooth muscle relaxation. PGE_1 also dilates the arterioles, thereby increasing blood flow into the penis. The tunica albuginea between the corpora cavernosa is highly perforated, allowing blood and pharmacological agents to pass easily from one corpus to the other. Therefore, the rush of blood engorges both corpora cavernosal sinusoidal spaces and creates an erection for a controlled period of time. After an injection with alprostadil, the patient can expect to obtain an erection within 5–20 min, the duration of which is approximately 30 min. The erection is immediate and will occur whether or not sexual stimulation is present, although subsequent sexual stimulation will enhance the effects.

Administration

- Alprostadil is usually started at a dose of 1.25 μg in patients with normal vascular symptoms and 2.5 μg for older patients or those with vascular compromise.
- Doses can be prescribed up to 20 μg.
- After retracting the foreskin, the patient holds the penis firmly in his non-dominant hand and injects slowly into the side of the shaft of the penis with the syringe perpendicular to the skin, taking care not to hit any of the large subcutaneous veins (which are usually visible).
- Once the needle is removed, firm pressure is applied to the injection site, and the drug is massaged gently throughout the shaft of the penis for approximately 30·s.
- Sometimes patients find it helpful to walk around the room, to increase blood flow.

The initial injection should be given by a medical professional demonstrating the sterile technique and monitoring the response to the injected agent. It is also helpful for the partner to be present, especially as it is often the partner who will carry out the injection, helping to make it seem an acceptable part of the normal lovemaking act. The erection should be monitored for rigidity and duration, and if this is adequate the patient can be taught to self-administer. Once the patient can confidently self-inject with a satisfactory technique, they should be prescribed a supply for home injection.

Side-effects and contraindications

Despite the treatment's proven efficacy, there has always been a very high drop-out rate associated with this type of treatment. Treatment failure or dropout occur in approximately 80% of patients within the first 12 months of usage [23]. Discomfort from injection, lack of spontaneity and inadequate erectile function are the usual reasons reported by patients for ceasing treatment.

Penile pain is thought to be due to the result of the acidity of the injection fluid, and the speed of the injection therapy is important, with slower injections (60 s) causing less pain than fast injections (5 s) [24]. With regard to the risk of priapism, patients should be warned that injection-induced erections often do not subside immediately after ejaculation as do normal erections, and may persist for an hour or two in some cases. However, if an erection lasts for more than 4 h, patients must seek immediate medical attention. Delayed treatment of prolonged erection can result in corpus cavernosum smooth muscle fibrosis from ischaemia, and therefore permanent and complete loss of erectile function.

On the positive side, there are relatively few contraindications to the use of intracavernosal injection therapy. However, due to the risk of priapism, patients with haematological abnormalities such as leukaemia, sickle-cell disease and significant coagulation problems should not be treated by this method and patients with poor manual dexterity must rely on their partners for injection.

Response rates

Provided the proper technique is used, up to 74% of patients achieve an erection satisfactory for intercourse [25].

Summary of intracavernosal injection therapy

Advantages
- Effective in up to 80% of men
- Good success rates if patient well motivated

- Suitable for most men with ED
- Few contraindications and drug interactions

Disadvantages
- Technique is too 'clinical' for some patients and their partners
- Lack of spontaneity
- Can be uncomfortable
- Patients need to be trained in the technique as manual dexterity and eyesight need to be adequate
- Risk of priapism
- May cause fibrosis in the corpora cavernosa

TRANSURETHRAL DRUG APPLICATION
Mode of action

Intraurethral delivery of alprostadil (Medicated Urethral System for Erection—MUSE®) provides a less invasive alternative to intracavernosal injection. Following micturition (a small amount of urine in the urethra helps the pellet to dissolve), a narrow (1.4 mm) pellet of synthetic PGE_1 is inserted with the aid of an applicator directly into the male urethra 15 min before intercourse. The drug quickly dissolves on insertion and blood vessel interconnections between the corpora cavernosa and the corpus spongiosum facilitate transurethral delivery. The increasing blood flow into the corpora leads to an erection, which usually lasts for 30–60 min.

Administration

- Available in concentrations of 125, 250, 500 and 1000 µg PGE_1.
- The dose used is 50 times higher than for the intracavernous route because a significant amount of the drug will enter the general circulation and never reach the corpora cavernosa.
- Efficacy can be increased by massage and using a constriction band at the base of the penis, which is applied prior to administration of the pellet.
- MUSE can be used up to twice daily.

Side-effects and contraindications

Although complications such as priapism and penile fibrosis are less common than after alprostadil given by penile injection, MUSE does seem to have a higher incidence of other side-effects, of which discomfort and tenderness are the most commonly reported. In one study by Porst [26], penile pain or burning was reported by 31% of the MUSE users compared with 10.6% of the intracavernous injection users. MUSE was also associated with dizziness, sweating or hypotension, although no patients receiving intracavernous injection experienced these symptoms. Although 80% of the drug is absorbed from the male urethra within 10 min of application, vaginal discomfort and itching can occur in the female partner. MUSE is not recommended for use with pregnant partners, as levels of PGE_1 in the ejaculate might induce labour (PGE_2 is used in pessary form to induce labour).

Efficacy

- Efficacy seems less easy to predict than with the intracavernosal route.
- 43% efficacy with MUSE vs. 70% with the intracavernosal injection therapy has been reported [26].

Summary of transurethral drug application

Advantages
- No needles involved
- Few contraindications, so acceptable for most men
- Efficacy seen in 27–66% [27,28] of men

Disadvantages
- Conflicting evidence of efficacy
- 30% incidence of penile pain [28]
- Must be inserted post-micturition
- Partners can complain of vaginal irritation
- Patients need to be taught how to use the technique—requires dexterity
- Risk of priapism (low)

VACUUM CONSTRICTION DEVICES

Medical literature suggests that vacuum pumps were first used to enhance penile function as early as the late 1800s. In 1917, the vacuum constriction device was patented by Dr Otto Lederer and acceptance of this management approach has increased with the development of the modern vacuum constriction device in 1982. Currently many companies manufacture vacuum constriction devices, providing patients and doctors with a large selection of models from which to choose.

Manufacturers of vacuum constriction devices

Dacomed Co.	NuMedTec Inc
Osbon Medical Systems Ltd	Post-T-Vac

Mentor	Mission Pharm
Vetco	Encore

Mode of action

The dynamics of a vacuum-assisted erection differ greatly from that of a phar-macological induced erection, in that there is no relaxation of the smooth mus-cle. There is some debate in terms of the exact physiological process that occurs when the vacuum is created around the penis. It has been suggested that the arterial inflow is actually unchanged, that venous outflow is reduced and the increase in penis diameter is due to blood collecting between the corpora and the skin. Others have found that there is an increase in arterial inflow. However, presumably the corpora cannot expand greatly as their smooth muscle remains contracted, although intracavernosal pressure does increase. The constriction ring, once applied, reduces both the arterial inflow and the venous outflow.

Administration

- Composed of three main parts:
  (i) a cylinder with one open end into which the penis is inserted
  (ii) a vacuum pump that is operated by hand or battery
  (iii) a constriction ring
- The penis is placed into the cylinder and the cylinder is pumped to produce a vacuum.
- The vacuum should be applied for approximately 6 min.
- Many manufacturers recommend pumping for 1–2 min, releasing pressure, and then resuming pumping for 3–4 min.
- Once an erection is produced, the constriction ring is slipped (off the cylinder) onto the base of the penis to maintain the erection.
- The ring should not be worn for more than 30 min or else the penis may suffer severe ischaemic damage.

Side-effects and contraindications

One of the main advantages of the vacuum device is that almost anyone can use it, with the exception of a few men with severe Peyronie's disease whose penile deformities are sufficiently severe not to allow insertion of the penis into the cylinder. The device should also be used with caution in men with bleeding or clotting disorders, as they run the risk of significant penile bruising, often at the site of the constriction ring.

In terms of side-effects, these are usually mild and do not require medical treatment, although partners often notice a reduction in penis skin tempera-ture and the penis can look slightly cyanosed, with distended veins. Additionally, the penis may pivot at its base, so the partner or patient may need to stabilize the penis during intercourse. The biggest cause of men dropping out from treatment with the device is the complaint that using a device can be cumbersome and interrupts sexual relations. Therefore this treatment is most suited to men with steady partners.

Efficacy

- Vacuum devices produce an erection in 92% of patients, regardless of the underlying cause of ED [29].
- Although some studies have reported success rates as low as 26% [30], it is only really men with severe corporal fibrosis who may have a poor response to therapy.

The success rate is probably mostly dependent on factors such as the enthusiasm of the instructing physician, the comprehensive nature of the training and the amount of time and encouragement given to the patient.

Summary of vacuum constriction devices

Advantages
- Suitable for most men with ED
- Very effective in most men
- Few contraindications
- Side-effects are usually very minor
- Suitable for long-term use

Disadvantages
- Lack of spontaneity/cumbersome
- Partners sometimes complain the penis feels cold
- Intercourse is limited to 30 min—if erections are maintained beyond this period there is a risk of ischaemia
- Vacuum-induced erections can feel uncomfortable
- The penis pivots at its base

SURGICAL TREATMENT FOR ED

Surgery may be considered in the case of certain conditions, or if all other treatment options have failed, are unacceptable or are contraindicated. There are a variety of surgical options available.

Penile prostheses

The majority of patients for whom a penile prosthesis is an option have probably suffered physical damage to the corpora, rendering other treatments ineffective. It is debatable whether patients with psychogenic ED should be considered for prosthesis, given that there is some evidence that these patients can have a higher complication rate and tend to be less satisfied with their prosthesis than men with organic disease. However, there have been cases where men have failed or refused to consider other treatments and this remains the only option.

Prostheses are either semi-rigid or inflatable. Semi-rigid prostheses are non-adjustable and consist of a pair of paired siliconized polyethylene cylinders, which are inserted directly into the corpora cavernosa. There are no postoperative mechanical problems associated with this method.

Inflatable devices consist of paired cylinders within the penis, connected to a reservoir and a pump that is put in the testicular sac. The pump moves fluid from the reservoir to the cylinders and vice versa, causing on-demand inflation and deflation of the cylinders. These devices are expensive and technically more difficult to implant. Future versions will have a remote control device similar to a garage door opener.

Side-effects and contraindications

The primary complication of surgical implantation is postoperative infection, which occurs in 1–10% of patients [31]. Infection can cause penile erosion, reduced penile sensation and auto-inflation. As infections can be difficult to treat, to avoid these further complications removal of the device may be required, although this occurs in less than 3% of infected patients. As infection is more common in diabetic patients it is particularly important to optimize glycaemic control several weeks before surgery in these patients.

Before any surgery is undertaken, patients must receive proper counselling and understand that the prosthesis will not improve libido and that the penis may not be as rigid as previously expected, and may even be shorter in length. The patient should also be aware that once surgery has been performed, none of the oral agents or vacuum devices will work in the future because of the changes to the penile architecture.

Response rates (in terms of satisfaction with treatment)

- 66–92% in patients [31]
- 60–80% in partners [31]

Advantages
- Can be used when other treatment options have failed or are contraindicated
- High success rate
- Provides a one-off solution

Disadvantages
- Higher incidence of complications than with medical treatment
- Possible mechanical malfunction of the prosthesis
- May require replacement at later date
- Risk of infection
- Penile size decreases
- Cost

VASCULAR SURGERY

Very occasionally it can be proven beyond doubt that ED is due to poor arterial inflow or abnormal venous drainage. On the rare occasions when this diagnosis can be made, the following surgical options are available.

Ligation of venous incompetence

Ligation of the deep dorsal vein of the penis is performed to increase venous outflow resistance in the corpora cavernosa, usually in men with a congenital abnormality in the cavernosal smooth muscle or tunica albuginea—the outcomes for such a procedure are usually poor.

Arterial revascularization surgery for arterial or venous abnormalities

Arterial revascularization is indicated in patients with arterial lesions in whom there is no significant atherosclerosis or atherosclerotic risk factors. Results of this surgery vary widely but are generally poor.

TESTOSTERONE THERAPY

Testosterone therapy with injections or patches is only indicated in men whose loss of libido/ED is due to hypogonadism (unless hypogonadism is due to a pituitary tumour), and should only be prescribed in patients with documented low testosterone levels. Testosterone deficiency is a rare cause of ED. It is important to repeat any random test sample at 9 a.m. to confirm the diagnosis.

Testosterone therapy is complex and specialist advice is advisable. It is administered orally or in the form of intramuscular injection or skin patches—implants are also available.

1

KEY POINTS

- ED is a very common condition, affecting up to 52% of men aged 40–70 years.
- There are a variety of ED treatments available including: oral therapy, intracavernosal injection therapy, transurethral drug application, the vacuum constriction device and psychosexual therapy.
- Sildenafil is the recommended first-line therapy for the majority of ED patients.

REFERENCES

1 Perttula E. Physician attitudes and behaviour regarding erectile dysfunction in at-risk patients from a rural community. *Postgrad Med J* 1999; **75**: 83–5.

2 Feldman HA, Goldstein I, Hatzichristou DG, Krane RJ, McKinlay JB. Impotence and its medical and psychosocial correlates: results of the Massachusetts Male Aging Study. *J Urol* 1994; **151**: 54–61.

3 Dunn K, Croft P, Hackett G. Sexual problems: a study of the prevalence and need for health care in the general population. *Fam Pract* 1998; **15**: 519–24.

4 Aytac IA, McKinlay JB, Krane RJ. The likely increase in erectile dysfunction between 1995 and 2025 and some possible policy consequences. *BJU Int* 1999; **84**: 50–6.

5 Kirby RS, Holmes S, Carson C. *Male Erectile Dysfunction*. Oxford: Health Press, 1997.

6 Boolell M, Allen MJ, Ballard SA *et al*. Sildenafil: an orally active type 5 cyclic GMP-specific phosphodiesterase inhibitor for the treatment of penile erectile dysfunction. *Int J Impot Res* 1996; **8**: 47–52.

7 Morales A, Gingell C, Collins M, Wicker PA, Osterloh IH. Clinical safety of oral sildenafil citrate (Viagra™) in the treatment of erectile dysfunction. *Int J Impot Res* 1998; **10**: 69–74.

8 Kloner RA, Brown M, Prisant LM, Collins M, Sildenafil Study Group. Effect of sildenafil in patients with erectile dysfunction taking antihypertensive therapy. *Am J Hypertens* 2001; **14**: 70 3.

9 Goldstein I, Lue TF, Padma-Nathan H *et al*. Oral sildenafil in the treatment of erectile dysfunction. *N Engl J Med* 1998; **338**: 1397–404.

10 Conti CR, Pepine CJ, Sweeney M. Efficacy and safety of sildenafil citrate in the treatment of erectile dysfunction in patients with ischemic heart disease. *Am J Cardiol* 1999; **83**: 29C–34C.

11 Rosen R, Shabsigh R, Menza M *et al*. The efficacy and safety of Viagra (sildenafil citrate) for the treatment of erectile dysfunction in men with comorbid depression. *Presented at 1st International Consultation on Erectile Dysfunction*, Paris, France, July 1999.

12 Rendell MS, Rajfer J, Wicker PA, Smith MD. Sildenafil for treatment of erectile dysfunction in men with diabetes. *JAMA* 1999; **281**: 421–6.

13 Fowler C, Miller J, Sharief M, for the Sildenafil Study Group. Viagra (sildenafil citrate) for the treatment of erectile dysfunction in men with multiple sclerosis. 124th Annual Meeting of the American Neurological Association, 1999, Seattle, WA, USA.

14 Giuliano F, Hultling C, El Masry W *et al*. Randomised trial of sildenafil for the treatment of erectile dysfunction in spinal cord injury. Sildenafil Study Group. *Ann Neurol* 1999; **46**: 15–21.

15 Data on file. Radical prostatectomy and TURP. Pfizer Ltd.

16 Heaton JP, Morales A, Adams MA, Johnston B, el-Rashidy R. Recovery of erectile function by the oral administration of apomorphine. *Urology* 1995; **45**: 200–6.

17 Mulhall JP, Bukofzer S, Edmonds AL, George M. An open-label, uncontrolled dose-optimization study of sublingual apomorphine in erectile dysfunction. *Clin Ther* 2001; **23**: 1260–71.

18 Von Keitz AT, Stroberg P, Bukofzer S, Mallard N, Hibberd M. A European multicentre study to evaluate the tolerability of apomorphine sublingual administered in a forced dose-escalation regimen in patients with erectile dysfunction. *BJU Int* 2002; **89**: 409–15.

19 Dula E, Bukofzer S, Perdok R, George M, the Apomorphine SL Study Group. Double-blind, crossover comparison of 3 mg apomorphine SL with placebo and with 4 mg apomorphine SL in male erectile dysfunction. *Eur Urol* 2001; **39**: 558–64.

20 Heaton JP. Characterising the benefit of apomorphine SL (Uprima) as an optimised treatment for representative populations with erectile dysfunction. *Int J Impot Res* 2001; **13** (Suppl. 3): S35–S39.

21 Klotz T, Sachse R, Heldrich A *et al*. Vardenafil increases penile rigidity and tumescence in erectile dysfunction patients; a RigiScan and pharmacokinetics study. *World J Urol* 2001; **19**: 32–9.

22 Patterson B, Bedding A, Jewell H, Payne C, Mitchell M. Dose-normalised pharmacokinetics of tadalafil (IC351) administered as a single dose to healthy volunteers. In: *4th Congress of the European Society for Sexual and Impotence Research*, 2001, Rome, Italy.

23 Kirby RS, Kirby MG, Farah RN. *Men's Health*. Oxford: ISIS Medical Media, 1999.

24 Gheorghiu D, Godschalk M, Gheorghiu S *et al*. Slow injection of prostaglandin E1 decreases associated penile pain. *Urology* 1996; **47**: 903–4.

25 Wagner G, Saenz de Tejada I. Update on male erectile dysfunction. *BMJ* 1998; **316**: 678–82.

26 Porst H. Transurethral alprostadil with MUSE (medicated urethral system for erection) vs intracavernous Alprostadil—a comparative study in 103 patients with erectile dysfunction. *Int J Impot Res* 1997; **9**: 187–92.

27 Fulgham PF, Cochran JS, Denman JL *et al*. Disappointing initial results with transurethral alprostadil for erectile dysfunction in a urology practice setting. *J Urol* 1998; **160**: 2041–6.

28 Padma-Nathan H, Hellstrom WJG, Kaiser FE *et al*. Treatment of men with erectile dysfunction with transurethral alprostadil. *N Engl J Med* 1997; **336**: 1–7.

29 Witherington R. Vacuum constriction device for management of erectile impotence. *J Urol* 1989; **141**: 320–3.

30 Gilbert HW, Gingell JC. Vacuum constriction devices: second-line conservative treatment for impotence. *Br J Urol* 1992; **70**: 81–3.

31 Eardley I, Sethia K, Dean J. *Erectile Dysfunction. A Guide to Management in Primary Care*. London: Mosby-Wolfe Medical Communications, 1998.

CHAPTER 2

Government Initiatives in Men's Health

'THE GENDER GAP'

Men are twice as likely to die before the age of 65 than women—the average life expectancy of men in the UK is 73.9 years compared with 79.2 years for women. No matter how often these statistics are quoted, the shock and the mystery remain; since the same modern medical technology and advanced treatments are available to all people regardless of gender, why are men still dying younger?

For many years it was believed that this 'gender gap' must be due to some intrinsic difference in overall disease susceptibility between the sexes—a trend that is set from birth, because death rates are greater in men than in women for each age group throughout life. Boys are more likely to be born prematurely and infant mortality is about 20% higher for boys than girls. Between the ages of 10 and 50 years, men are more prone to accidents and violence (in 1992 deaths from injury and poisoning accounted for 52% of deaths in the 15–39 years age-group in men). This is usually explained by men being notoriously higher risk takers than women—for example, driving cars too fast and participating in dangerous contact sports (Fig. 2.1).

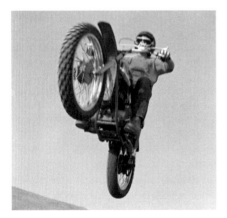

Fig. 2.1 Men as risk-takers.

Disturbingly, the incidence of mortality in young men is increasing. In the last three decades, male youth suicide rates have nearly doubled and suicide is now the most frequent cause of death in men between the ages of 15 and 24 years. Increasing confusion over the male's role in society and rising unemployment levels are believed to be possible reasons for this. Unemployment can severely affect a man's sense of well-being, self-esteem and purpose. Statistics show that long-term illness is 40% higher in unemployed men compared with unemployed women.

Although these statistics offer some explanation for the gender difference in life expectancy in terms of accidental death and suicide, there is another simple unavoidable fact—men simply do not take as good care of their health as women do. On average, men consult their GP four times less often than women (one-third less likely) and even then usually only because their partner has told them to. This is true even when women's gynaecological and reproductive health reasons to attend their surgery are excluded. Not presenting to the doctor at the first sign of symptoms means that a diagnosis may not be reached until a disease is at an advanced or even incurable stage. Men's lack of concern for their health may go some way towards explaining the high mortality rates associated with certain conditions in men.

CAUSES OF DEATH

So what are the most common causes of death in the nation's men? Table 2.1 sheds some light on the matter [1].

Table 2.1 Relative causes of male deaths in the UK [1].

Disease	Per cent of male deaths
Coronary heart disease	24
Stroke	8
Other cardiovascular diseases	8
Lung cancer	10
Prostate cancer	4
Colorectal cancer	3
Other cancers	15
Respiratory disease	9
Injuries and poisoning	7
All other causes	12

Cardiovascular disease

Cardiovascular disease (CVD) is the leading cause of mortality in the United Kingdom—it accounts for over 235 000 deaths a year. Coronary heart disease (CHD) alone accounts for 26% of deaths among men [1].The cost of CVD is not only great in terms of human life—CHD costs the NHS about £1600 million a year. Hospital care for people who have CHD accounts for about 54% of these costs [1]. The total cost to the NHS for treating heart disease, stroke and related illness is a staggering £3.8 billion each year [1].

Cancer

Cancer is the second most frequent cause of male mortality in the UK—in 1990 over 136 000 men in the UK were diagnosed with cancer, and in 1994 over 82 000 men died of the disease. Prostate cancer is the most frequently diagnosed cancer in western men. In the UK, 21 000 men are diagnosed with prostate cancer each year and 10 000 men die as a result. Testicular cancer is the most frequently occurring cancer in men aged 20–45, with recent trends suggesting an increase, particularly in the western world [2].

However, many cancers, if not preventable, are at least potentially curable if identified early enough. Sadly, most men remain reluctant to take steps to prevent the development of malignant disease. For example, a study of male students across Europe found that 87% had never examined their testicles [3]. Although recent and increasing media interest has hopefully raised the profile of this disease amongst young men and encouraged self-examination, education is desperately needed in most other areas of men's health to encourage men to take responsibility for their own health. More than £60 million is spent annually on screening for breast and cervical cancer in women, yet little is being done to target the prevention and early detection of cancer in men.

GOVERNMENT INITIATIVES

Education is vital to convince men (and women) to take more responsibility for their health. Primary healthcare in the UK and around the world is undergoing a number of fundamental changes. There is increasing recognition of the importance of lifestyle and environmental factors in staying healthy and maintaining quality of life. Effective health promotion and controlling of risk factors are key to the prevention and early identification of most conditions, issues that are increasingly important to the government. The WHO/UNICEF Alma-Ata declaration of 1978, which was subsequently reflected in the *Health of the Nation* report, has led to increasing interest in health promotion and disease prevention.

The *Health of the Nation* improvement targets prioritized by key health areas

- Heart disease and stroke
- Cancers
- Mental illness, depression, anxiety and related consequences, such as suicide
- Sexual health, particularly containment of HIV/AIDS
- Accidents

OUR HEALTHIER NATION

The Department of Health (DoH) set out the framework for a new health strategy for the UK in a white paper, *Saving Lives: Our Healthier Nation*, in 1999. Its twin aims were to improve the health of the nation as a whole by increasing the length of people's lives and the number of years people spend free of illness, and to improve the health of the worst-off in society and narrow the health gap. It acknowledges that loss of good health is no longer about blame but about opportunity and responsibility. It highlights that individuals can find it hard to make a difference, but when they are supported by the primary healthcare team, who work together with families, local agencies and communities, deep-seated problems can be tackled. Well Man clinics play a small but very important part in this scenario—the aim being to persuade men to take more responsibility for their own health. *Our Healthier Nation* set out clear targets for improvements in four priority areas (Table 2.2).

NATIONAL SERVICE FRAMEWORKS

National Service Frameworks (NSFs) were introduced in 1998 as a new DoH initiative to create national standards for healthcare provision, determine

Table 2.2 Healthcare targets set by the 1999 White Paper, *Our Healthier Nation*.

Healthcare area	Target
• Heart disease and stroke	• To reduce the death rate from heart disease and stroke-related illness among people aged under 65 years by at least one-third
• Accidents	• To reduce accidents by at least one-fifth
• Cancer	• To reduce the death rate from cancer amongst people aged under 65 years by at least one-fifth
• Mental health	• To reduce the death rate from suicide and undetermined injury by at least one-sixth

strategies for care delivery and establish performance markers to monitor progress. Each NSF represents a 10-year funded programme and so far four NSFs have been published—mental health, coronary heart disease, older people, and diabetes (part published). NSFs for renal services and children are due soon. Separate frameworks exist for Scotland, Wales and Northern Ireland. The NSFs for diabetes and CHD are of particular relevance to erectile dysfunction (ED).

NSF FOR CHD

The DoH has already set out in *Our Healthier Nation* their ambition to reduce by two-fifths the death rate from heart disease, and related illnesses such as stroke, in those aged under 75 by 2010. The *NSF for CHD* published in March 2000 requires GPs to identify all patients with established CHD or stroke, document their risk factors and offer treatment. More than 90% of practices now have active CHD registers (and it was stipulated that practices should have set up disease registers to identify CHD patients by April 2001). The NSFs obviously have implications for GPs in terms of increased workload. Therefore, there is a need to maximize the skills of nurses and to recruit more GPs and nurses.

Managing ED can play a large role in helping GPs to meet targets set out in the *NSF for CHD*. As will be discussed in some depth in Chapter 3, ED can be a marker for CVD, sometimes when there are no other symptoms. Proactive identification of ED in patients should prompt the primary healthcare team to investigate other risk factors for CVD, hence enabling earlier diagnosis of underlying CVD and identification of those patients who are likely to develop CVD in the future. This would go some way to enabling the first four standards of the NSF to be fulfilled, as these are all related to the proactive identification of CVD and coronary risk factors.

1   The NHS and partner agencies should develop, implement and monitor policies that reduce the prevalence of coronary risk factors in the general population.
2   The NHS and partner agencies should contribute to a reduction in the prevalence of smoking in the local population.
3   GPs and primary care teams should identify all those with established CVD and offer them comprehensive advice and appropriate treatment to reduce their risks.
4   GPs and primary care teams should identify and treat those who have not yet developed symptoms but who are at significant risk of developing CVD.

NSF FOR DIABETES IN ENGLAND

The number of people with diabetes in the UK will have doubled between 1995 and 2010—making it one of the fastest growing threats to health in the UK today. At the time of writing, the *NSF for Diabetes* was still awaiting publication.

So far, 12 standards have been published in England (published in December 2001). The first standard focuses on prevention. The NHS aims to develop, implement and monitor strategies to reduce the risk of developing Type 2 diabetes in the population as a whole. Standard 2 shows that early identification of people with diabetes is also a priority—the charity Diabetes UK estimates that around a million people in England, mostly aged 40 and over, have diabetes without knowing. As ED is a risk factor for diabetes, proactive identification of ED could lead to earlier identification of diabetes in men, hence helping to fulfil standard 2.

Standard 2. Early identification of people with diabetes

> Increase awareness of risk factors, symptoms and signs of diabetes, and increase screening of those at recognized risk.

A STRATEGY FOR SEXUAL HEALTH (Fig. 2.2)

The importance of sexual health is becoming increasingly recognized on the UK healthcare agenda, being a key issue that concerns the majority of the population. The government's consultation document, *The National Strategy for*

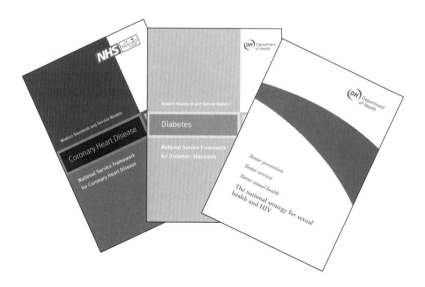

Fig. 2.2 DoH documents relevant to the management of ED.

Sexual Health and HIV (for England), published in July 2001, is the first time that there has been a national approach to sexual health. This National Strategy outlines opportunities for developing sexual health services in primary care, and aims to:

- Improve access to healthcare services, information and support for all who need them
- Reduce inequalities in sexual health
- Improve health, sexual health and well-being
- Provide a new system of organizing care into different levels of practice

The strategy document sets out a definition of sexual health that is a welcome statement about the range of determinants of sexual health. However, the consultation paper focuses mainly on the prevention and treatment of sexually transmitted infections and HIV, and contains little on ED. Although the strategy does make some important and welcome suggestions about the treatment of sexual dysfunctions such as ED, it could be argued that these recommendations do not go far enough.

In October 2001, the DoH decided to continue the restrictions for GP prescribing of NHS treatments for ED established in July 1999 (Health Service Circular 1999/148). These guidelines (called Schedule 11) prevent GPs from prescribing NHS treatments to patients whose ED is not caused by a specified problem. This means that men whose ED is caused by diabetes or severe pelvic injury, for example, can be treated by GPs on the NHS, while men whose ED is caused by CVD or depression cannot. The guidelines stand in stark contrast to the DoH's repeatedly stated aim of encouraging men to take better care of their health and to report problems to a health professional, and reinforce the notion that men's health issues are not taken as seriously by the NHS as they should be. This makes it more difficult to encourage men to pay more attention to any health problem they may suffer from. This directly contradicts the government's sexual health strategy, which states that:

'Sexual health is an important part of physical and mental health .... Essential elements of good sexual health are equitable relationships and sexual fulfilment with access to information and services to avoid the risk of unintended pregnancy, illness or disease.'

The Schedule 11 prescribing restrictions need to be reviewed by the DoH to eliminate the restrictions on access to NHS treatments for erectile dysfunction.

IMPLEMENTING THE SEXUAL HEALTH STRATEGY

Services must be implemented to encourage men affected by erectile dysfunction and other sexual dysfunctions to seek help, particularly through non-traditional methods of service delivery such as drop-in clinics, websites and telephone information services. In order for these services to be implemented effectively, education of healthcare professionals in the importance of proactive ED identification and management is essential. Nurses have a vital role to play in this, as they frequently run clinics where patients have a greater likelihood of having ED, e.g. diabetes and hypertension clinics. Well Man clinics also offer the healthcare professional an ideal opportunity to ask men proactively about their erectile function as part of a general health check.

2

REFERENCES

1   *British Heart Foundation statistics database*, 1997/2002.

2   Moore RA, Topping A. Young men's knowledge of testicular cancer and testicular self-examination: a lost opportunity? *Eur J Cancer Care* 1999; **8**: 137–42.

3   Wardle J, Steptoe A, Burckhardt R *et al.* Testicular self-examination: attitudes and practices among young men in Europe. *Prev Med* 1994; **23**: 206–10.

Identification and Management of Risk Factors

3

RISK FACTORS FOR CARDIOVASCULAR DISEASE

In order to identify and arrest the onset of disease effectively, it is important to target the people who are most at risk of developing the disorder. For example, coronary heart disease (CHD) is a chronic condition that has many risk factors, many of which are also risk factors for erectile dysfunction (ED). Table 3.1 outlines some of the risk factors healthcare professionals should look out for when trying to detect the likelihood of the patient developing CHD or ED.

It seems that the pattern for future development of cardiovascular disease (CVD) could be set from an early age.

- Only 55% of boys aged 2–15 years and 39% of girls are active for the recommended 1 h 5 days or more a week [1].
- 15% of teenagers and over 12% of children are now clinically obese, which is a time bomb for public health [2].

Table 3.1 Risk factors for cardiovascular disease and their incidence in the UK [1].

Risk factor	Incidence in men	Incidence in women
Overweight and obesity	46% overweight Further 17% obese	32% overweight Further 21% obese
Raised blood pressure	41%	33%
Raised blood cholesterol	66%	67%
Diabetes	3%	3%
Smoking	28%	26%
Alcohol consumption over daily recommended limits	38%	21%
Physical activity < 30 min × 5 days/week	63%	75%

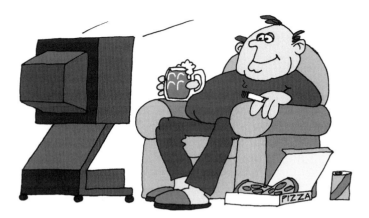

Diabetes

Diabetes also significantly increases the risk of CVD and CHD—middle-aged men with diabetes are around five times more likely to die of CVD than men without diabetes [1]. Since 1991, the incidence of diabetes has increased by around two-thirds in men and a quarter in women. Currently, about 1.4 million people in the UK have been diagnosed with diabetes, and this number is set to double by 2010. It has been estimated that there are currently 1 million people whose diabetes has not yet been diagnosed [3].

Hypertension

Hypertension is one of the most common conditions managed in primary care. Using the 'new' definition of systolic or diastolic pressures of at least 140 or 90 mmHg, respectively, 41% of men and 33% of women are hypertensive [1]. The number of men who are not receiving treatment for their hypertension remains disturbingly large—according to the British Heart Foundation, just over 80% of men with hypertension are not treated [1].

Obesity

An increasing proportion of men have a body mass index (BMI) of > 25, with 46% of men being classified as overweight and a further 17% classified as obese [1]. A man with a BMI of 22–23 is about half as likely to suffer from CHD than a man with a BMI > 30 and he is eight times less likely to develop diabetes [4]. Aside from being a disease in its own right, obesity also leads to increased cardiovascular risk, insulin resistance, dyslipidaemia, hypertension and Type 2 diabetes.

  With so many men affected by ill health, in most cases largely self-inflicted through an unhealthy lifestyle, the time has never been better for the primary healthcare team to proactively identify these risk factors and target lifestyle intervention.

ED AS A MARKER

ED may be a marker for a number of conditions and should set warning bells ringing with every primary healthcare professional. A patient presenting with ED offers an opportunity for the primary healthcare team to detect their patient has, or is at risk of, not only CVD but a multitude of other concurrent conditions. Treatment improves the patients' sexual and psychological well-being, and facilitates the management of chronic illnesses earlier in the disease process. A study of 980 men seeking medical advice because of their ED [5] found that:

- 18% were also suffering from undiagnosed hypertension
- 16% had diabetes
- 15% had benign prostatic hyperplasia
- 5% had ischaemic heart disease
- 4% had prostate cancer
- 1% had depression

Many patients (and even doctors) may just want a 'quick fix' for their ED, and as the choice of treatment is not generally dependent on the underlying cause, the need for a full assessment might be mistaken as superfluous. Good medical practice means taking a holistic approach towards diagnosis before initiating treatment. For example, if a patient presented to a surgery with pain, the physician would not prescribe painkillers without locating the source and reason for the pain. The underlying cause of ED in the patient should be established and, where possible, treated before, or at the same time as, initiating therapy specifically for the ED.

RISK FACTORS FOR ED

As well as being a marker for other underlying conditions, ED is also a serious medical condition in its own right. It has its own set of risk factors or underlying conditions that should prompt the physician to question the patient about their sexual function. For effective ED management it is crucial to identify the diseases, psychosocial factors and other risk factors that may cause or maintain ED. Healthcare professionals must be vigilant in their proactive identification of ED, as it could be a new symptom of a previously diagnosed condition or the first presenting symptom of a previously undiagnosed condition [5,6]. The prevalence of underlying cardiovascular conditions in patients presenting with ED should provide the impetus to healthcare professionals to raise the subject of ED proactively.

To realize the full impact and implications of the important link between ED, CVD and other underlying pathologies, it is useful to examine the physiology and statistics with regard to the incidence of ED in relation to specific underlying conditions.

ED AND CVD
Prevalence of cardiovascular risk factors in patients with ED

It is estimated that between 39% and 64% of male patients with CVD suffer from ED [7]. CVD can generally be subdivided into four conditions—atherosclerosis, coronary artery disease (CAD), hypertension and peripheral vascular disease. Any of these four conditions can predispose the patient to developing ED. The Massachusetts Male Ageing Study found that after age-adjustment, men with heart disease, diabetes or hypertension are up to four times more likely to develop some degree of ED compared with men who do not suffer from these disorders.

Vascular endothelium—a starring role

The vascular endothelium provides the source of the critical association between ED and CVD, as it plays a vital role in regulation of the circulation (Fig. 3.1).

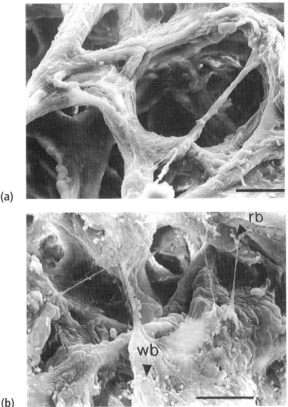

(a)

(b)

Fig. 3.1 Electron micrographs of (a) normal penile vascular endothelium and (b) the effect of diabetes in the rabbit. Note the ragged appearance of the endothelium and the deposition of red blood cells (rb) and white blood cells (wb) in diabetes. Micrographs courtesy of M. Sullivan.

Hypertension, ischaemic heart disease and hypercholesterolaemia can all lead to abnormalities of the vascular smooth muscle cells and the extracellular matrix. This endothelial cell dysfunction can precede the formation of atherosclerotic plaques and is common in CVD and diabetic patients [8]. Patients with diabetes have endothelial dysfunction and an increased risk of developing cardiovascular complications. Impaired endothelium-dependent vasodilatation via nitric oxide (NO) is also well documented in CAD and in conditions such as diabetes, hypertension and dyslipidaemia [9].

ED is a marker for disease progression

ED can also provide an important measure of CVD progression and severity. For example, patients with single-vessel ischaemic heart disease have firmer erections and less difficulty in obtaining an erection than those patients with two or three vessel disease [10], the penis thereby acting as a barometer of cardiovascular status.

Early identification of CHD risk

A study of a group of healthy men complaining of ED found that 60% had abnormal cholesterol levels, and > 90% showed evidence of penile arterial disease during Doppler ultrasound imaging [11] (Fig. 3.2). In another study it was discovered that 80% of asymptomatic males with ED displayed at least one risk factor for CVD. Patients who subsequently underwent coronary angiography were found to have significant CAD with over half diagnosed with multivessel disease [12]. Therefore, routine investigations into the ED patient's cardiovascular status can aid the identification of previously undiagnosed CVD.

PATHOPHYSIOLOGY OF ED IN CVD
Atherosclerosis (Fig. 3.3)

Disease of the vascular tree, from the aorta to the penile arteries, can cause ED by restricting the inflow of blood into the penis. As the narrow vessels of the penis may be more prone to blockage than the larger vessels of the heart, the atherosclerotic process may actually begin in the small penile arteries [12]. As the usual pattern is one of diffuse disease, it therefore follows that ED can be indicative of arterial disease elsewhere in the body.

Fig. 3.2 (a) Normal penile Doppler ultrasound. The cavernosal artery Doppler waveform is normal and peak systolic velocity (PSV) is over 35 cm/s. (b) Arterial insufficiency on penile Doppler ultrasound. Severely reduced cavernosal artery flow with PSV of only 11 cm/s. (c) Venous insufficiency on penile Doppler ultrasound. Normal systolic flow (PSV 35 cm/s) but end diastolic velocity (EDV) is elevated, with lowered resistance index, indicative of veno-occlusive failure. Doppler ultrasound images courtesy of J. Haworth, R. Jones and C. Gingell.

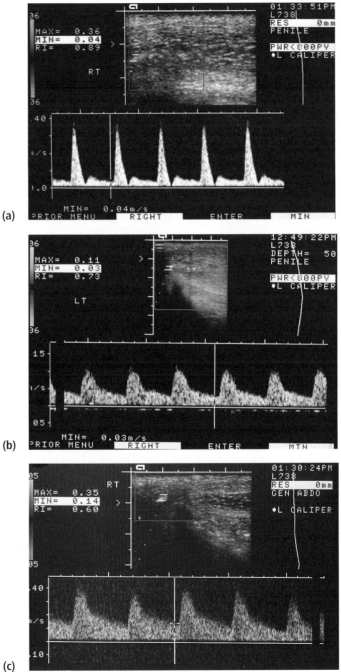

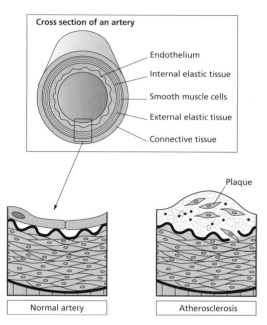

Fig. 3.3 Normal artery vs. atherosclerotic artery.

Venogenic causes of ED

Erectile function also depends on the veno-occlusive mechanism, which operates when the cavernosal tissue expands, compressing the emissary veins as they pass through the tunica albuginea, preventing blood from leaving the penis. If this mechanism fails, excess blood will leak out continuously from the penis through venous channels that have not shut down. This will clearly prevent an erection from reaching its full capacity and being maintained. Pathological causes of failure of the venous part of the veno-occlusive mechanism are very rare. It more commonly fails because of inadequate arterial flow, due to either organic or psychogenic factors. Possible causes of venous failure [13] are:

- Decreased smooth muscle content of the corpora cavernosa, with smooth muscle cells replaced by connective tissue.
- Decreased nerve stimulation.
- Decreased endothelial cell production of NO.
- Reduction in compliance of the extravenous drainage channels, due to ageing changes in the collagen of the tunica.

Hypertension

It has been found that ED is not only more prevalent in patients with hypertension than in an age-matched general population, it is also more severe in those with hypertension than in the general population.

- In men with hypertension, mild ED was found in 7.7%, moderate ED in 15.4% and severe in 45.2% [14].
- 60.9% of patients with hypertension and 77.9% of patients with both hypertension and diabetes admitted to ED problems [15].

Despite this evidence of a link between hypertension and ED, the physiological process is unclear. Some argue that the NO–cGMP-mediated haemodynamic mechanism of erection and the NO–cGMP-mediated pathway of vasodilation that play a vital role in blood pressure regulation are impaired in both ED and hypertension. However, it has been found that hypertension alone does not impair the penile-brachial index and arteriograms are normal in 91% of those cases. As incidence of ED can reach 100% in those with three or more arterial risk factors, the link between hypertension and ED could be simply that hypertensive patients have more additional risk factors of atherosclerotic disease [16].

The hypertensive patient's medication could play the biggest role in the development of ED. A series of studies [17–19] found that the incidence of ED in hypertensive patients ranged from 17% in patients with untreated hypertension to 25% (rising to 68%) in patients with treated hypertension. Antihypertensive drugs affect not only the blood pressure, but also the compliance of the erectile tissue, resulting in a functional venous leak, and impair erectile function as much as atherosclerotic changes of the vascular system secondary to the hypertension itself.

Previous myocardial infarction

A history of myocardial infarction (MI) is associated with the development of ED. Studies have found the incidence of ED to range from 44% to 64% in patients who have previously had an MI [7,17]. In this instance ED can occur as a result either of the general risk factors for CVD mentioned above which may have led to the MI (the ED may well have been present before the MI took place). In addition, psychogenic causes are significant post-infarct.

CVD and psychogenic ED

Sir William Osler (quoted by Garfield, 1976) [20] once said:

'It is so much more important to know what sort of a patient has a disease than what sort of a disease a patient has'.

Psychological problems and fears are particularly common in the CVD patient, and can be the main cause of their ED. For example, the post-MI patient or post-cardiac bypass surgery patient may fear that sexual activity will precipitate an MI. The healthcare professional must establish the underlying thoughts of the patient about his condition so that the appropriate advice and reassurance can be given to allay the patient's fears and concerns about the risks of resuming or initiating sexual activity. It is important not to forget that the partner may also be sharing and feeding these fears; therefore it is essential, wherever possible, to provide counselling to both the patient and his partner together as a couple. If ED is of mainly psychogenic cause, it is possible that following advice, reassurance and initial treatment, the patient may have a spontaneous return of their erections.

ED AND DIABETES

Awareness is gradually increasing that ED is a significant and common complication of diabetes. The cardiovascular and neurological complications associated with diabetes increase the risk of developing ED by a complex mechanism that interferes with the interaction between the endothelium and the smooth muscle cells.

Prevalence of ED in diabetic patients

- Over 50% of diabetic men have suffered from ED at some time, and as many as 39% suffer ED all the time [21].
- ED is estimated to occur in 30% of all diabetic men and at least 50% of male diabetics over 60 years old [18].

The onset of ED in diabetic men usually occurs gradually, and often 10–15 years earlier than in those without diabetes. The high rates of ED in men with diabetes are usually a result of vascular disease and neurological/autonomic dysfunction, and there is a striking degree of overlap between typical co-morbidities of diabetes and risk factors for ED:

- Peripheral neuropathy
- Vascular insufficiency
- Dysfunction of both the cavernosal endothelium and smooth muscle
- Poor glycaemic control
- Treated or untreated hypertension
- Low testosterone levels
- Obesity
- History of smoking

These risk factors are all significantly more common in diabetic subjects than in non-diabetic subjects [10,22]. As with CVD, because of this sharing of risk factors ED can also be a marker for diabetes.

Pathophysiology of ED in diabetic men

The greater the length of time the patient has diabetes and the concurrent metabolic indices of inadequate diabetes control (such as concentrations of blood glucose and glycated haemoglobin), the greater the risk of ED. Diabetes mellitus (DM) is associated with atherosclerosis of the large arteries, and it appears more frequently and at an earlier age than in non-diabetics. Atherosclerosis consequently also affects the penile and pudendal arteries, limiting the blood flow into the corpus cavernosum. Diabetic ED is also associated with microangiopathy, characterized by increased thickening of the capillary basement membrane, and other manifestations of diabetic vascular disease such as retinopathy, intermittent claudication and the risk of amputation.

Autonomic neuropathy is a major contributor to the high incidence of ED in diabetic men, as it initially affects small unmyelinated fibres which innervate the corpora cavernosa, leading to depletion of relaxant neurotransmitters within the penis (low intracavernosal NO synthase levels). It has also been shown that advanced glycation products in diabetes may also adversely affect NO signalling mechanisms within the corpora cavernosa [23]. As NO is needed to activate the cGMP to subsequently relax the corpus cavernosal smooth muscle, this can prevent intracavernosal blood pressure from rising to a level sufficient to compress the venous channels and hence stem emissary vein outflow. Therefore the erection is unable to be acquired or maintained. Smokers and men with testosterone deficiency also experience these low NO levels and may hence develop ED through a similar process to the diabetic patient.

Identifying diabetes in the ED patient

The primary care team should routinely test men who present with ED for diabetes, for the following reasons:

- ED is a marker for underlying diabetes.
- The cost of active case-finding in high-risk groups is likely to be less than that of caring for a more advanced patient with diabetes.
- There is a clear link between quality of blood glucose control and risk of diabetic complications.
- Therefore, removing psychological factors that could affect a patient's management of their blood glucose, such as ED, should be a priority in order to manage both the ED and the diabetes effectively [24].

To establish whether diabetes is the underlying cause in men with ED, dipstick testing alone is not adequate. It has been found that if the dipstick test alone is used to identify the presence of diabetes in men with ED, four out of five new cases of DM will be missed (80%) [25]. Fasting blood glucose should be undertaken to diagnose diabetes reliably in men with ED.

Type 2 diabetes often goes undiagnosed for many years and such patients are at increased risk of developing microvascular (retinopathy) and macrovascular complications (CHD, stroke, peripheral vascular disease). Fifty per cent of patients with diabetes have evidence of diabetic tissue damage at diagnosis [26]. Adequate glycaemic control reduces the risk of these complications. Glycaemic control measured using HbA$_{1c}$ predicts erectile function [27], and improved glycaemic control also leads to improved erectile function. In nurse-led ED clinics a fasting blood glucose assessment should be incorporated into the management protocol.

ED OF NON-VASCULAR CAUSE

Although ED is most commonly vascular in origin, as the cause of ED can be complex and multifactorial, it is important to be familiar with other possible contributing factors to the ED when planning the overall management of the patient.

Depression and ED

ED can be a symptom of depression as much as depression can be a symptom of ED. It is important to differentiate between the two, as treatment strategies may differ. Depression can either be reactive (caused by a specific event or situation such as bereavement, loss of job, etc.) or endogenous (occurs for no reason). Whatever the cause of the depression, ED may well be compounding the patient's negative feelings and in some instances may be the root cause of the depression. For many men the ability to maintain erectile function is a very important part of their life and so any reduction in this ability could have a negative impact on the patient's feeling of self worth and confidence. As previously discussed, antidepressant medication can also induce sexual dysfunction, with the incidence of ED varying from 1.9% to 92% [28].

There is also a three-way link between ED, CVD and depression. Depression can predict future cardiac adverse events in patients with CAD, and can even hasten mortality [29]. One explanation for this is that depressed patients may experience increased medical complications because of deficits in their ability to problem-solve, cope with challenges and comply with medical therapy and rehabilitation [30].

Neurogenic causes of ED

Any disease process or injury affecting the brain, spinal cord or pelvic nerves can cause ED (e.g. multiple sclerosis (MS), stroke, multisystem atrophy, spinal cord injury and tumours). Some studies have shown that 71% of men with MS [31] and 86% of men following stroke [32] have ED. ED most commonly occurs between 4 and 9 years after MS is diagnosed. However, the pathophysiological mechanisms will vary according to the site and type of neural damage.

Peripheral nervous system

Conditions affecting the cauda equina such as prolapsed intervertebral discs or tumours can interrupt the parasympathetic 'erectogenic' pathways to the pelvic plexi. In the same way, disease or damage to the parasympathetic nerves within the pelvis can also lead to ED. The most common cause of this damage is diabetes and injury following radical pelvic surgery.

Spinal cord and central nervous system

Spinal cord injury is more common among younger men and the frequency and form of any resulting ED is dependent on the severity and level of the injury. If the spinal cord injury is complete, and high, psychogenic erections do not occur, although many men do have reflex erections in response to direct genital stimulation. Men who have a lower spinal lesion may lose these reflex erections due to associated ischaemia of the lumbrosacral cord. However, with lesions below T12, the sympathetic pathways are still functional, and so psychogenic erections are still possible, although they are not present in all patients.

Surgery or trauma

Any extensive surgical procedure involving the pelvis or lower abdomen may lead to the inadvertent destruction of nerves or blood vessels that supply the corpora cavernosal bodies in the penis. For example, erectile dysfunction remains the most common problem following radical prostatectomy, with rates ranging from 100% to 10% depending on the experience of the surgeon, the frequency with which he or she performs the surgery, the nerve-sparing nature of the procedure, the stage of the disease, and the age and preoperative potency of the patient.

- Incidence of ED in patients with localized prostate cancer who have received radiotherapy is at least 26% [33].
- TURP (transurethral resection of the prostate) and bladder neck incision surgery can also result in ED, with incidence rates of 13.6% and 4.6%, respectively [34].

Trauma, irradiation or surgery involving the pelvic region frequently result in ED, usually through the inadvertent damage of nerves or arteries that supply the corpora cavernosa. In the case of TURP, diathermy damage to the cavernous nerves as they pass lateral to the prostate is the most likely cause of the ED. The incidence of ED is particularly high in men who undergo ileostomy or colostomy, as the associated change in body image can also lead to psychogenic ED.

Age-related changes

With increasing age, a number of changes occur in erectile function. The libido is decreased, penile sensitivity is diminished and it takes longer for a full erection to be achieved. In older men, the higher centres of the brain are less reactive to psychogenic stimuli such as fantasizing and audio-visual stimuli so that erections become more dependent on manual stimulation. Increased interaction between the couple, especially in terms of foreplay, is needed to achieve a satisfactory erection. There is a decrease in the frequency, duration and rigidity of nocturnal erections and an increase in the refractory period (the time from ejaculation to the next erection). This interval may range from 30 min in a young man to several days in an octogenarian, according to the work of Masters and Johnson.

Although some men presenting with ED appear to have no physical cause of their ED apart from their age, more commonly, there are also organic or psychogenic elements which reflect the increasing prevalence of risk factors in men as they grow older. For example, with increasing age there is a fall in testosterone levels, and vascular and structural changes within the penis. There may also be a psychological element involved. For example, if older men fail to recognize that they need longer to become aroused, this delay could lead to increased performance-related anxiety, which in turn could lead to a vicious circle, resulting in complete loss of erectile function. Although some men will choose to accept ED as a natural consequence of ageing and choose not to seek treatment for it, with the advent of less invasive treatments for ED increasing numbers of men are selecting to prolong their sexual careers.

Renal disease

Forty-five per cent of patients with chronic renal failure experience ED [35]. This figure increases by a further 35% following commencement of dialysis [35]. There are a number of pathophysiological processes which lead to the problem, including hyperprolactinaemia, hypogonadism, smooth muscle dysfunction due to circulating toxins, neuropathy and atherosclerosis. Conditions which result in renal failure such as diabetes mellitus may also add to the problem, as may the treatments used to treat the consequences of renal failure such as antihypertensives and renal dialysis.

Peyronie's disease and other structural abnormalities of the penis

As the structure of the fibroelastic vascular tissue of the trabecular spaces is a key factor in making an erection possible, any damage to this structure could potentially affect the erectile function. Changes in the smooth muscle cells of the vascular system and the trabecular spaces can result from several diseases (such as Peyronie's disease) as well as ageing.

Medications

Many prescription drugs are associated with ED (Table 3.2), although it must be remembered that these drugs may also be treating conditions that in themselves cause ED. Examples of this are hypertension and antihypertensives, depression and antidepressants, and dyslipidaemia and cholesterol-lowering drugs. Many 'recreational' drugs are also associated with ED. Although there is very little high-quality evidence to establish a link between ED and most of these drugs, if there is a strong relationship between the start of drug therapy and the onset of ED, this should be considered as highly indicative of an iatrogenic problem.

If medication is seen as being the main cause of the ED it would seem that the most obvious course of action is to remove or change the medication in the hope that the ED will spontaneously resolve without the need for further treatment. However, there is little evidence to confirm the effectiveness of reversing ED by a change in drug therapy. It has been found that changing hypertensive medication does not affect the systemic blood pressure level [36], suggesting a direct influence on the erectile tissue through possible effects on the central nervous

Table 3.2 Medications that can cause ED.

Cardiovascular drugs	Psychotropic drugs
Thiazide diuretics	Major tranquillizers
β-blockers	Anxiolytics and hypnotics
Calcium antagonists	Tricyclic antidepressants
Centrally acting agents	Selective serotonin reuptake inhibitors
methyldopa	
clonidine, reserpine	**Endocrine drugs**
ganglion blockers	Anti-androgens
Digoxin	Oestrogens
Lipid-lowering agents	LHRH analogues
ACE inhibitors	Testosterone
Recreational drugs	**Others**
Alcohol	Cimetidine and ranitidine
Marijuana	Metoclopramide
Amphetamines	Carbamazepine
Cocaine	
Anabolic steroids	
Heroin	

system, parasympathetic nervous system or hormonal balance. Altering or ceasing medication may be appropriate if a careful history is taken and there is a very definite strong link between the start of therapy and the onset of ED, although it should be noted that following change or removal of medication it would be expected that any improvement in ED would be likely to occur within 2–4 weeks.

Before any modifications to drug treatments are undertaken, it is vital to consider the impact of modifying drug treatment on the underlying disease they are being used to treat, and to take into consideration whether there is an alternative medication that could be used to treat the underlying condition but would not lead to ED, e.g. in the instance of a patient receiving β-blockers for the treatment of hypertension, α-blockers or an angiotensin II inhibitor could be used as an alternative option. In some instances a change in medication, despite the beneficial effect this might have on the patient's erectile function and psychological well-being, may not be in the patient's best interests in terms of their overall health. For example, β-blockers are prognostically beneficial post-MI and in patients with heart failure, so should not be stopped abruptly or without consideration of the overall risk to the patient. It should also be considered that the ED may be due to the condition being treated, e.g. hypertension, ischaemic heart disease or atherosclerosis, rather than the drugs used.

KEY POINTS

- ED may be a marker for a number of conditions including CVD, diabetes and depression.
- The underlying cause of ED in the patient should be established, and vascular risk factors identified, before initiating therapy specifically for the ED.
- Routine investigations into the ED patient's cardiovascular status can aid the identification of previously undiagnosed CVD.
- Fasting blood glucose should be undertaken to reliably diagnose diabetes in men with ED.
- Many prescription drugs are associated with ED.

REFERENCES

1 British Heart Foundation statistics database, 2002.
2 Reilly JJ, Dorosty AR. Epidemic of obesity in UK children. Lancet 1999; **345**: 1874.
3 Diabetes UK. http://www.diabetes.org.uk/home.htm (last accessed 1 August).
4 Baker P. Real Health for Men. London: Vega, 2000.
5 Curkendall SM, Jones JK, Glasser D, Goehring E. Incidence of medically detected erectile dysfunction and related diseases before and after Viagra (sildenafil citrate) [Abstract 324]. Eur Urol 2001; **37** (Suppl. 2): 81.

6   Kloner RA. Erectile dysfunction and cardiovascular risk factors. *Hosp Pract (Off Ed)* 2001; **36**: 41–4, 49–51.

7   Bortolotti A, Parazzini F, Colli E, Landoni M. The epidemiology of erectile dysfunction and its risk factors. *Int J Androl* 1997; **20**: 323–34.

8   Kirby M. Lipid management can reduce CHD in diabetes. *Best Practice* 2001; March: 31–2.

9   Quyyumi AA, Dakak N, Mulcahy D *et al.* Nitric oxide activity in the artherosclerotic human coronary circulation. *J Am Coll Cardiol* 1997; **29**: 308–17.

10   Greenstein A, Chen J, Miller H *et al.* Does severity of ischemic coronary disease correlate with erectile function? *Int J Impot Res* 1997; **9**: 123–6.

11   Billups K, Friedrich S. Assessment of fasting lipid panels and doppler ultrasound testing in men presenting with erectile dysfunction and no other medical problems. In: *95th Annual Meeting of the American Urology Association,* 2000, Atlanta, USA.

12   Pritzker MR. The penile stress test: a window to the hearts of man? (Poster). In: *72nd Scientific Session of the American Heart Association,* 1999, Atlanta, USA.

13   EDIPC. *Erectile Dysfunction in Primary Care: Module 1.* Pfizer Ltd, 1998.

14   Burchardt M, Burchardt T, Baer L *et al.* Hypertension is associated with severe erectile dysfunction. *J Urol* 2000; **164**: 1188–91.

15   Giuliano F, Leriche A, Jaudinot E *et al. Erectile Dysfunction in Patients with Diabetes and/or Hypertension.* Rome: ESSIR, 2001.

16   Virag R, Bouilly P, Frydman D. Is impotence an arterial disorder? A study of risk factors in 440 impotent men. *Lancet* 1985; **1**: 181.

17   Wabrek AJ, Burchell RC. Male sexual dysfunction associated with coronary heart disease. *Arch Sex Behav* 1980; **9**: 69–75.

18   Alexander WD. Sexual function in diabetic men. In: Pickup JC, Williams G, eds. *Textbook of Diabetes,* 2nd edn. Oxford: Blackwell Science, 1997: 59.1–59.12.

19   Bulpitt CJ, Dollery CT, Carne S. Change in symptoms of hypertensive patients after referral to hospital clinic. *Br Heart J* 1976; **38**: 121–8.

20   Garfield CA. Foundations of psychosocial oncology: the terminal phase. *Front Radiat Ther Oncol* 1976; **2**: 180–212.

21   Hackett GI. Impotence—the most neglected complication of diabetes. *Diabetes Res* 1995; **28**: 75–83.

22   Kannel WB, Wilson PW, Zhang TJ. The epidemiology of impaired glucose tolerance and hypertension. *Am Heart J* 1991; **121**: 1268–73.

23   Seftel AD, Vaziri ND, Ni Z *et al.* Advanced glycation products in the human penis: elevation in diabetic tissue, site of deposition, and possible effect through iNOS or eNOS. *Urology* 1997; **50**: 1016–26.

24   Diabetes Control and Complications Trial Group. Effect of intensive diabetes management on macrovascular events and risk factors in the Diabetes and Complications Trial. *Am J Cardiol* 1995; **75**: 894–903.

25   Sairam K, Kulinskaya E, Boustead GB, Hanbury DC, McNicholas TA. Prevalence of undiagnosed diabetes mellitus in male erectile dysfunction. *BJU Int* 2001; **88**: 68–71.

26   UK Prospective Diabetes Study Group. Overview of 6 years' therapy of type II diabetes: a progressive disease. *Diabetes* 1995; **44**: 1249–58.

27 Romeo JH, Seftel AD, Madhun ZT *et al.* Sexual function in men with diabetes type 2: association with glycaemic control. *J Urol* 2000; **163**: 788–91.

28 Balon R, Yeragani VK, Pohl R, Ramesh C. Sexual dysfunction during antidepressant treatment. *J Clin Psychiat* 1993; **54**: 209–12.

29 Roose SP. Sexual activity and cardiac risk: is depression a contributing factor? *Am J Cardiol* 2000; **20**: 38F–40F.

30 Glassman AH. Depression and the course of coronary artery disease. *Am J Psychiat* 1998; **155**: 4–11.

31 Goldstein I, Siroky MB, Sax DS, Krane RJ. Neurological abnormalities in multiple sclerosis. *J Urol* 1982; **128**: 541–5.

32 Agarwal A, Jain DC. Male sexual dysfunction after stroke. *J Assoc Physicians India* 1989; **37**: 505–7.

33 Flanigan RC, Patterson J, Mendiondo O *et al.* Complications associated with pre-operative radiation therapy and iodine-125 brachytherapy for localised prostatic carcinoma. *Urology* 1983; **22**: 123–6.

34 Roehrborn C. *Standard Surgical Interventions.* Oxford: ISIS Medical Media, 1996.

35 Abram H, Hester L, Sheridan W, Epstein G. Sexual functioning in patients with chronic renal failure. *J Nerv Mental Dis* 1975; **160**: 220–6.

36 Newman RJ, Salerno HR. Sexual dysfunction due to methyldopa (letter). *Br Med J* 1974; **4**: 106.

CHAPTER 4

Guiding the Patient

THE IMPORTANCE OF SEX

4

There is no doubt that for most men, sex is a very important part of their life. During adolescence, boys compete to lose their virginity; young men judge themselves on the size, firmness and staying power of their erections, and their number of sexual partners; and older men can worry about being able to achieve an erection at all.

The ability to attain and maintain an erection is integral to a man's sense of well-being and can be crucial in maintaining a good relationship with his partner [1]. An inability to 'perform' poses a direct threat to a man's core belief in himself and can be a very traumatic event.

Although it is normal for sexual interest and capacity to decline with advancing age, it becomes an issue when this is not proportional to the needs of the patient or his partner. More than 80% of men and 60% of women aged between 40 and 80 years feel that sex is an important part of their lives, and at least 57% of men and 51% of women of this age still have sex regularly (at least 1–6 times per week) [2]. Embarrassment, fear and ignorance can result in a significant number of men not approaching their doctor when their erections fail and so deny themselves the opportunity for a fulfilling sex life well into their old age.

THE IMPACT OF ERECTILE DYSFUNCTION

Most people's lives are split into a number of domains, such as work, family, friends and relationships. A problem in one of these domains can also affect other domains. This is particularly true in the case of men and their ability to have sex—if a man is able to achieve his sexual goals, he will feel satisfied with his life overall. If there is a sexual aspiration–achievement gap, decrease in sex satisfaction can lead to decreased overall life satisfaction [3]. Erectile dysfunction (ED) has a profound effect on all aspects of a patient's psychological and social functioning, including his capacity to work, maintain social and family roles and sustain self-esteem [4]. It has been shown that quality of life can be substantially diminished by ED [3,5,6].

If the patient has a serious underlying medical condition, this may affect his quality of life even further. For example, it has been shown that diabetic men with ED have a greater reduction in quality of life than non-diabetic men with ED [7]. As discussed in Chapter 3, the loss of self-esteem and anxiety associated with ED in diabetic men may also decrease a patient's motivation to manage his diabetes properly, increasing the risk of additional complications of the underlying condition [8].

The benefits of treating ED extend beyond simply restoring sexual function—effective treatment of ED can also improve the patient's quality of life [9]. Treatment has been shown to improve health-related quality of life as well as sexual function in many men [10,11].

IMPACT ON RELATIONSHIPS

The impact of ED on the relationship of a couple can be, without question, huge. In one study of men with ED and their partners, nearly three-quarters of women said that the man usually initiated sexual activity [12]. However, a man with ED may withdraw from sexual activity completely, fearing that he may be unable to 'perform'. The man may eventually avoid any form of contact that could be seen as a prelude to something that he feels unable to participate in. This can place a huge strain on the relationship, because neither partner is now receiving any kind of affection at all. The following disturbing statistics were found in a study of men with ED and their partners [13]:

- Only 10% of couples had experienced any sexual kissing or caressing in the 4 weeks before presentation.
- Almost half of the couples had not experienced *any* sexual activity for 2.5 years.
- Almost 84% of men rated sexual intercourse as important, compared with only 20% of women. However, both men and women overestimated the importance that their respective partners placed on intercourse.
- There was clinical evidence of urogenital atrophy in a third of women (over 46 years).

A survey of 3693 men seen by RELATE counsellors found that one in four men who required these services had some degree of ED [14]. In another study, 27% of couples in which the man had a sexual problem had significant marital problems [15]. An Impotence Association survey in 1997 found that 20% of men with ED had experienced broken relationships as a result of their condition [16]. Furthermore, 8% of partners had considered ending the relationship because of ED.

Table 4.1 Impotence Association survey results (2000 & 2001) [17].

Effect on quality of life and relationships	Proportion of men (%)
Depressed or made to feel depressed by ED	32
Worried and anxious	65
Lacking confidence	62
Negative feelings caused by ED	46
Relationship difficulties	35
Worsened relationship	28
Breakdown in relationship	7
Stopped forming relationships	12

BROACHING THE SUBJECT OF ED

- Only one in 10 men with ED aged between 18 and 59 years seeks medical attention for ED [18].
- Nearly 60% of men with ED have not previously received treatment for their ED [17].
- Of these, 69% wish to be treated and 58% want the physician to discuss the subject of their erections.
- Despite regular clinic visits, only 33% of diabetic patients with ED had discussed the problem with their GP [7].
- Although patients with hypertension visit physicians regularly for antihypertensive treatment, many do not receive treatment for ED (33%) [19].
- Only 14% of men with diabetes and 8% of men without diabetes had been asked by their physician about sexual problems [20].
- However, nearly 50% of men with diabetes and 47% of men without diabetes felt that they should routinely be asked about their sexual health [20].

These statistics highlight first that a disturbingly high number of men suffer needlessly with their ED without seeking treatment, and second that men would like to be asked about their erectile function by a healthcare professional. Considering the increase in awareness of male sexual health in the past few years and the ever-increasing number of treatment options available, why are so few men seeking help?

WHY AREN'T PATIENTS INITIATING DISCUSSIONS ABOUT SEX?

The main reason why men would rather suffer in silence than consult their doctor is embarrassment. In one study, 44% of men with ED failed to tell their urologist and, of these, 71% cited embarrassment as the main reason for not raising the topic [21].

- Up to 71% of patients think that the doctor will dismiss any concerns about sexual problems.
- Patients view sexual activity as a 'luxury' rather than a serious health concern, or think that their doctor feels that way [22].
- Many patients do not associate ED with their medical condition—for example, research has shown that fewer than half of men with diabetes and ED associate their erectile problems with their diabetes and only one in five blames the diabetes medication for the ED [7].
- Elderly couples who are now experiencing sexual problems were raised in an era when sex was a taboo topic.
- Men may feel ashamed or humiliated at having to ask for help for a condition that they may feel compromises their masculinity.

Embarrassment—how to recognize it

The concept of embarrassment is very important in healthcare. It deters patients from seeking treatment and adopting 'healthy' behaviour and it deters staff from broaching topics such as sexuality. But what exactly is embarrassment? Elias [23], writing in the 1930s, argued that embarrassment is a fairly recently developed emotion. Fear of physical attack was once the predominating emotion in humans, when life-threatening events were a daily occurrence. In more recent times, the absence of such threats has led to these emotions being increasingly replaced by fear of shame and embarrassment.

Situations relating to embarrassed feelings are typically unpleasant and the trigger usually stems from a concern about making an undesired impression. Signs of embarrassment include reduced eye contact, increased body movement, speech disturbances and blushing. Embarrassment can also be infectious, so it is important that healthcare staff take care not to appear embarrassed by either the subject area or indeed the patient's discomfort. Otherwise, the patient may become even more embarrassed himself and be unwilling or unable to discuss his problem.

Other reasons for avoiding the topic

- The patient is not bothered by his ED.
- Misinformation about available treatment options.
- He seldom seeks medical advice or treatments for any reason.
- The partner may be afraid of treatment side-effects or simply have a lack of interest in resuming sexual activity.
- Cost of ED treatment.

WHY AREN'T HEALTHCARE STAFF INITIATING DISCUSSIONS ABOUT SEX?

Research suggests that healthcare staff can also have difficulties discussing sexuality.

- 47% of adult patients have never been asked by their primary care physicians whether they have sexual relationships [24].
- Although nearly three-quarters of doctors said that they routinely asked 80–100% of their male patients about ED, doctors actually initiated discussion about ED in only 17% of men with hypertension, 18% with diabetes and in only 30% of those aged over 65 [25].
- If the subject of erectile function is discussed in a consultation, it is most often raised by the patient (85% of the time) [26].
- Prescribing policy related to Schedule 11 causes confusion to both doctors and patients.

4

There are many reasons for doctors and nurses not taking the initiative in discussing sexual problems. Although everyone is familiar with basic history taking, uncertainty on how to obtain information on a patient's sexual function in a non-threatening way is a common explanation. Other factors include lack of time, perceptions about the age, gender and culture of the patient, and belief that the patient will initiate discussions.

Surveys have shown that patients actually want and expect to be asked about sexual problems. In one study, 91% of patients thought that it was appropriate for their physicians to take a sexual history [27]. Many patients who find it difficult to initiate the discussion are in fact desperate to be asked and saved the embarrassment of raising the subject themselves. Given the doctor or nurse's perceived position of authority, it is his or her place to put the patient at ease and raise this important subject in a comfortable and professional manner.

HOW TO BROACH THE ISSUE: PROACTIVE IDENTIFICATION OF ED

Creating the best environment for a discussion of sexuality starts before the patient even enters the doctor's office.

- Be completely comfortable with personal attitude towards sexual issues before discussing those of the patient.
- Understand normal sexual functioning, sexual responses and psychosexual development, as well as any cultural, religious or ethical implications.
- Be familiar with the full range of human sexual expressions and behaviours, in order to communicate effectively and understand the patient's point of view.

- Never judge or provide moral advice when responding to the patient's sexual questions or concerns, no matter what the patient says.
- Do not make assumptions about a patient's sexuality; for example, ask 'Who are the most important people in your life?' or 'Are you sexually active with men, women or both?'

If healthcare staff feel uncomfortable about the prospect of discussing erectile function, they should remember that ED may be the first presenting symptom in men with unidentified heart disease. Thus, routine sensitive questioning about ED provides the team with another opportunity to assess and identify undiagnosed cardiovascular disease (CVD) and diabetes.

Recognize the patient's approach

When talking about embarrassing subjects, patients are often vague and try to talk around the subject. It is vital to clarify exactly what the patient is trying to communicate. If the patient gives short, terse answers, this should not be interpreted as rudeness or unwillingness to talk, but rather as embarrassment or even underlying depression. It is also important to accept that some patients may never overcome their discomfort with discussing their erections, especially with a woman.

It is also common for patients to talk about other, unrelated health matters first, before mentioning their sexual problem. If this occurs, it must be decided which health matter needs the most or immediate attention, and the patient may need to be asked back for a longer consultation later. However, if it has been a struggle for him to bring up the topic of ED once, he may not attend another appointment unless he is given definite signals that his condition is to be taken seriously.

PRACTICAL TIPS FOR DISCUSSING SENSITIVE ISSUES

The key to encouraging a patient to talk is trust. Trust can be facilitated through effective listening skills and a non-judgmental, accepting and empathetic attitude. The ability to recognize behavioural and cultural cues is invaluable in the healthcare setting, because these skills help to demonstrate the empathy and professional expertise needed to encourage patients to discuss their problems.

In terms of the practicalities of ensuring that the atmosphere, environment and conversation put the patient at ease, the following factors need to be taken into consideration.

Environment

It is often better if the first consultation is with the patient alone, in case he needs to reveal information that he does not want his partner to know about (e.g.

extramarital affairs); after the initial assessment, the patient's partner should be involved in any further discussions.

- Use a relaxing and private room.
- Close the door after the patient and put a sign on the door asking not to be disturbed.
- Sit at the side of the desk so that there is no table acting as a barrier—this also allows the patient's body language to be observed.

Body language

Observing body language provides an indication of how nervous or embarrassed the patient is, and can help the doctor or nurse to adjust the style of questioning in a bid to put the patient at ease. Signs to look out for include the following:

4

- Use of hands and arms, e.g. fidgeting, defensively crossing arms or protectively holding a bag or briefcase on his lap.
- Position in the chair—is the patient slumped in a depressed way, sitting tautly bolt upright or sprawling in a relaxed manner?

The doctor or nurse needs to be sure to look the patient straight in the eye, because the patient might interpret any avoidance of eye contact as embarrassment and may therefore feel ill at ease himself. Female staff, especially young women, should be taught how to establish a relationship with open discussion. Few older men feel comfortable discussing their erections with a healthcare professional young enough to be their daughter or even granddaughter, so the woman needs to ensure that the atmosphere remains professional but relaxed and that the patient feels comfortable. If the patient is still reluctant to discuss sexual issues, consideration should be given to enlisting the support of a colleague.

Time

One of the greatest gifts that a patient can be given is time to discuss his problems. Even though time is usually limited, especially in a busy practice, efforts should be taken to ensure that the patient does not feel he is being rushed, as he may read this as a sign of lack of interest. A simple silence provides the patient with the opportunity to expand on a point and reassures him that the doctor or nurse is not rushing him and wants to hear what he has to say.

If time really has run out, the patient should be told that the importance of his problem justifies a longer appointment to get to the root cause and identify successful treatment options. Another appointment should be arranged there and then so that he does not lose confidence and motivation to discuss his problem.

Terminology

The language used by healthcare professionals to describe and explain medical terms to patients is crucial to ensure that both parties fully understand each other. Patients may be unsure whether to use colloquialisms (fearing that they may cause offence) and so may try to express their problem in medical terms. However, patients frequently get the meanings wrong, which can cause confusion for both parties. For example, patients can use 'impotence' to mean failure to get an erection, failure to maintain an erection, infertility or even premature ejaculation. Repetition of the patient's last word or phrase, especially if it is an emotive term, encourages the patient to elaborate on what he is trying to say and can help to avoid misunderstanding.

Both the use of language that the patient is likely to understand, and the avoidance of such terms (because they are emotionally charged) can cause problems in obtaining an accurate history. Some patients feel embarrassed hearing colloquialisms and would prefer to discuss their sexual problem in more professional, medical terms; others may not understand medical terms and would feel more comfortable talking in a language that they use every day. The healthcare professional needs to use careful judgement to decide whether it would be more appropriate to use 'street language' or medical terms, or as is more often the case, a mixture of both. The decision usually rests on the person's background, age and gender.

TAKING A SEXUAL HISTORY

If the healthcare professional considers that the patient may have a problem with ED, a full sexual history should be taken.

- Explain the purpose of the questions to the patient.
- Explain that some questions may be personal.
- Reassure the patient of complete confidentiality—this is particularly important if the patient wants to divulge details such as extramarital affairs.
- Normalize the situation to encourage the patient to relax and express information.
- Reassure the patient that his responses and concerns are not unusual and that there are no 'stupid' questions.
- If the patient is unwilling to talk about intimate matters despite encouragement, ask 'Are you sure you don't have any questions?' and then let the subject rest until another appointment.

'Do you have any questions?' is probably the most important question to ask, because patients frequently respond by asking about the one thing that concerns them most. Some patients come to a consultation with one burning question but, if not given the opportunity to ask that question, may leave without an answer.

Asking open questions

Open questions are vital if the real root of a sexual problem is to be uncovered. The first few questions are critical for putting the patient at ease, reassuring him that any problems are normal and encouraging him to discuss his sexual function. Introducing the subject as a problem that commonly coexists with heart disease or diabetes and explaining that asking about ED is a routine part of that assessment is perhaps the most appropriate approach.

Sample questions to encourage the patient

> • 'It is quite common for men with diabetes to experience problems with getting an erection. Is this a problem you've experienced? Is it a problem you would like to do something about?'
>
> • 'Some men have difficulties resuming sexual activity [after bypass surgery, after a heart attack, if they are taking medication]. Have you experienced any problems?'

If it is felt that the patient does have ED, supplementary questions can then determine the extent and exact nature of the problem. For example, the next question could be 'Do you have erections when you wake up in the morning, very first thing?'. This establishes the clinical tone and hopefully projects clinical interest in the man's erectile function, rather than a judgement about his performance.

ADDRESSING RELATIONSHIP ISSUES

ED and its management affect not only the patient, but also his partner, whose needs therefore must also be addressed during the consultation process.

Identifying relationship issues

If the partner is present during the consultation, valuable clues about the couple's relationship can be gleaned. Is there any expression of physical affection or touching? Is one person overly protective, irritated or stressed? It is helpful to discover any psychogenic factors that may be affecting the patient or his partner.

> • A strict upbringing and strong religious beliefs can often have a huge effect on a sexual relationship.
> • Unemployment or threat of it can lead to anxiety and subsequently ED.
> • Retirement can lead to loss of self-esteem in either the patient or partner, which can also affect sexual performance.
> • After children leave home it is common for sex drive to be increased—any disparities between the couple's sexual desires and needs should be addressed.
> • Marital dysfunction or even boredom can also be a major cause of ED.
> • Previous sexual abuse can impact on relationships.

However, some issues need to be addressed with care when the partner is present. For example, the patient may be reluctant to talk about masturbation in front of his partner, or he may want to talk about extramarital affairs. Although ED can significantly impact on a homosexual relationship, there is a lack of research in this area and therefore this chapter focuses on the female partner.

Impact of relationship issues on ED management

There are many ways in which the partner, or the relationship as a whole, can affect the treatment outcome. If a couple has not had sexual contact for many years, it may be very difficult for them to resume sexual intercourse when erectile function is restored. Sex therapy may be desirable to facilitate resumption of sexual activity and provide a non-threatening environment in which the partner can express concerns; for example, the partner may have sexual problems herself that need to be addressed. There is a high prevalence (62%) of sexual disorders in the female partners of men with ED—including primary and secondary orgasmic dysfunction, vaginismus, dyspareunia and impaired sexual interest; in only 8% of cases did these dysfunctions precede the onset of the ED. This indicates that the partner's ED can lead to sexual dysfunctions in the woman [28].

Female sexual dysfunction [29]

- A woman's motivation to be sexual often stems from intimacy needs.
- Multiple biological and physical factors, including those linked to diabetes (in women), can cause breaks in a woman's sex response cycle.
- The motivation to be sexual again can be weakened by a negative outcome such as loss of orgasmic experience associated with more severe forms of diabetic neuropathy, or a partner's sexual dysfunction.

In some instances, a woman's sexual problem may be hidden behind her partner's erectile disorder, which may contribute to the development of ED. If this is the case, the woman's problem is often revealed only when her partner's erectile function is re-established. This can result in outcome failure even if treatment restores her partner's erectile function (if the desired outcome is sexual intercourse). In some instances, to ensure successful treatment, the woman may need to be treated before the therapy for ED is initiated. Because the man may not volunteer this information or may not be aware of it, this is another reason why it is so important to include the woman in discussions about the sexual relationship.

The effect of the sexual experience on the woman's self-esteem is an important consideration when selecting a treatment option. A woman generally wants to have some sense that the man's erectile response is due to her—if her partner has to use a pump or inject himself in order to have sex, she may feel that she has failed sexually because he cannot obtain a 'normal' erection. It is therefore not surprising that the woman might be resistant if her partner attempts to use these methods to induce erection, although this can be a confusing response for the man who has finally managed to gain an erection.

This is less of a problem with oral medication, because the erectile response is generated only in the presence of sexual stimulation. Thus, the woman is involved in the arousal process and can feel that she has a role, although some women might still feel fundamentally undesired because their partner has to take a pill to become aroused. Because of these fears, it is essential that the woman understands her role in the arousal process and realizes that her partner's reliance on mechanical or medicinal means to obtain an erection is due to a physical problem rather than her undesirability.

The partner's reaction to the man's ED can, especially in the case of a psychogenic cause, play a huge part in perpetuating the cycle. If the partner makes the man with ED feel inadequate, guilty or ashamed of his inability to obtain an erection, through defensiveness and their own feelings of inadequacy, this can only compound the problem. It is therefore important that restoring erectile function is not the only objective—it is essential to address interpersonal and intrapersonal factors, all of which may have precipitated or maintained the sexual problem.

INVOLVING THE PARTNER

Unfortunately, partners are often neglected in the process of establishing the cause of the ED and appropriate management strategies. It is therefore not surprising that some partners have, consciously or unconsciously, affected a potentially successful outcome of treatment of their partner's ED. Partners therefore need to be given the opportunity to discuss their concerns and any problems that they may have.

Partners, like the patients themselves, may be concerned about the cause of the ED as well as any side-effects of treatment. In addition, if the man has heart disease, both he and his partner may be worried about the effect of sexual activity on his heart. Efforts must be taken to ensure that the patient and partner are counselled appropriately and that all concerns are put into perspective. The safety of ED treatments and sexual activity in those with CVD is discussed in more depth in Chapter 5.

The partner should also be asked whether big life changes, such as the menopause or a hysterectomy, have affected the way that she perceives herself, and the partner needs to be reassured that it is common for women to feel less feminine or attractive to their partner after these events. The healthcare professional should also explain that depression, irritability and emotional and social withdrawal are all normal reactions to ED for both partners.

One study found that clinicians may alter their diagnosis and treatment options as much as 58% of the time if they take the partner's views into account [30].

HEALING THE RELATIONSHIP: COUNSELLING IN PRIMARY CARE

Although most cases of ED have an organic cause, the contribution of psychogenic factors and the role of counselling in patients whose ED has a significant psychogenic cause should not be underestimated.

- The patient with severe psychogenic ED may require a greater level of counselling expertise than is usually provided in the general practice setting.
- Sex therapy can address poor verbal and non-verbal communication between the patient and his partner.

Psychotherapy, as well as being very rewarding, is also time consuming and requires a significant level of expertise and experience; this is the domain of a specialist counsellor. There are usually three types of psychosexual therapy.

Exclusive psychosexual therapy

- Six to ten sessions.
- With the patient alone or the couple together.
- Cognitive, behavioural and interpretative therapies facilitate an understanding of and a strategy for overcoming problems.
- Follow-up procedures essential.

Sex therapy in conjunction with medical treatment

- Ensures that treatment is being used and is satisfactory for both partners.
- Addresses psychological, emotional and relationship factors that remain a concern.

Information/education on sexual activity

- For patients who simply need permission, guidance and confidence to recommence a sexual activity that is mutually satisfying.
- On some occasions, a specialist will need to be involved.

The following tables (Erectile Dysfunction in Primary Care, EDiPC) provide a list of factors to look for when deciding who would benefit from psychosexual therapy. These include early experiences that are likely to make a person vulnerable to developing difficulties at a later stage, events or experiences associated with the initial appearance of ED, and factors that sustain the problem.

When referring a patient for psychosexual therapy or counselling, it is helpful to have attempted to identify which of these components have been or are still important drivers in causing the condition.

Predisposing factors [31]

Inadequate sexual information
Sexual beliefs
Impact of culture on sexual expectations, fears and performance
Disturbed family relationships
Traumatic early sexual experiences
Insecurity in sexual role

Precipitating factors [31]

Relating to men
Generalized anxiety
Specific sexual anxieties (fear of failure, pregnancy, HIV, meeting women's sexual demands)
Depression
Addictive behaviour
High levels of stress, particularly relating to life events
Ageing (perception and related fears/distortions, rather than physical process)
Psychological reaction to organic factors
Inability to express sexual needs and preferences
Random failure

Relating to the partner or couple
Sexual dysfunction or difficulties in the partner (vaginismus, inhibited sexual drive/ arousal)
Infidelity
Discord in the relationship
Fear of intimacy or commitment
Poor communication
Reaction to pregnancy and childbirth
The partner's own ageing process, which may include menopausal difficulties

Maintaining factors [31]

Inadequate sexual information throughout the sexual lifecycle
Reinforced performance anxiety/anticipation of failure
Guilt and shame
Impaired self image
Loss of attraction and desire between partners
Restricted foreplay
Poor communication between partners
Relationship conflict/breakdown
Psychiatric disorders

4

KEY POINTS

- A man's quality of life can be substantially diminished by ED, and if the patient has a serious underlying medical condition, this may affect his quality of life even further.
- ED can also have a very negative impact on the relationship.
- As ED can also be a marker for underlying chronic conditions such as CVD and diabetes, both patients and healthcare professionals must become more proactive in raising the subject of ED during consultations.
- To encourage a successful treatment outcome, the partner should be involved wherever possible.

REFERENCES

1 MORI. *Attitudes Towards Erectile Dysfunction: a Survey of Men Aged 40+*. 1998.
2 Pfizer. *The Pfizer Global Study of Sexual Attitudes and Behaviours*. Pfizer Inc., 2002.
3 Fugl-Meyer AR, Lodnert G, Branholm IB, Fugl-Meyer KS. On life satisfaction in male erectile dysfunction. *Int J Impot Res* 1997; **9**: 141–8.
4 Zurowski K, Kayne H, Goldstein I. *The Social and Behavioral Costs of Organic Impotence.* Abstract presented at the annual meeting of the American Urological Association, San Francisco, 1994.
5 Litwin MS, Nied RJ, Dhanani N. Health-related quality of life in men with erectile dysfunction. *J Gen Intern Med* 1998; **13**: 159–66.
6 Jonler M, Moon T, Brannan W *et al.* The effect of age, ethnicity and geographical location on impotence and quality of life. *Br J Urol* 1995; **75**: 651–5.
7 Hackett GI. Impotence—the most neglected complication of diabetes. *Diabetes Res* 1995; **28**: 75–83.
8 Cummings MH, Alexander WD. Erectile dysfunction in patients with diabetes. *Hosp Med* 1999; **60**: 638–44.
9 Quirk F, Giuliano F, Peña B, Smith MD, Hockey H. Effect of sildenafil (Viagra™) on quality-of-life parameters in men with broad-spectrum erectile dysfunction [Abstract 998]. *J Urol* 1998; **159** (Suppl. 5): 260.

10 Fujisawa M, Sawada K, Okada H *et al.* Evaluation of health related quality of life in patients treated for erectile dysfunction with Viagra (sildenafil citrate) using SF-36 score. *Arch Androl* 2002; **48**: 15–21.

11 Giuliano F, Pena BM, Mishra A, Smith MD. Efficacy results and quality-of-life measures in men receiving sildenafil citrate for the treatment of erectile dysfunction. *Qual Life Res* 2001; **10**: 359–69.

12 Carroll JL, Bagley DH. Evaluation of sexual satisfaction in partners of men experiencing erectile failure. *J Sex Marital Ther* 1990; **16**: 70–8.

13 Riley A, Riley E. Behavioural and clinical findings in couples where the man presents with erectile disorder: a retrospective study. *Int J Clin Pract* 2000; **54**: 220–4.

14 McCarthy P, Thoburn M. *Psychosexual Therapy at RELATE: a Report on Cases Processed Between 1992 and 1994.* RELATE Centre for Family Studies and RELATE Marriage Guidance, 1996.

15 Catalan J, Hawton K, Day A. Couples referred to a sexual dysfunction clinic: psychological and physical morbidity. *Br J Psychiat* 1990; **156**: 61–7.

16 *Impotence Association Survey.* London: Taylor Nelson AGB Healthcare, 1997.

17 *Impotence Association Survey.* London: 2000 and 2001.

18 Laumann EO, Paik A, Rosen RC. Sexual dysfunction in the United States: prevalence and predictors. *JAMA* 1999; **281**: 537–44.

19 Burchardt M, Burchardt T, Baer L *et al.* Hypertension is associated with severe erectile dysfunction. *J Urol* 2000; **164**: 1188–91.

20 Nicolosi A, Glasser D, Brock G *et al.* Diabetes and sexual function in older adults: results of an international survey. *Br J Diabetes Vasc Dis* 2002; **4**: 336–9.

21 Baldwin KC, Ginsberg PC, Harkaway RC. Underreporting of erectile dysfunction among men with unrelated urologic conditions. Abstract presented at Annual Meeting of the American Urological Association, Atlanta, 2000.

22 Marwick C. Survey says patients expect little physician help on sex. *JAMA* 1999; **281**: 2173–4.

23 Elias N. *The Civilising Process,* Vol. 1, *The History of Manners.* Oxford: Basil Blackwell, 1976.

24 Mathews WC, Linn LS. AIDS prevention in primary care clinics: testing the market. *J Gen Intern Med* 1989; **4**: 34–8.

25 Perttula E. Physician attitudes and behaviour regarding erectile dysfunction in at-risk patients from a rural community. *Postgrad Med J* 1999; **75**: 83–5.

26 Broekman CPM, Van Der Werff JJ, Ten Bosch MD. The patient with erection problems and his general practitioner. *Int J Impot Res* 1994; **6**: 59–65.

27 Ende J, Kazis L, Ash A *et al.* Measuring patient's desire for autonomy: decision making and information seeking preferences among medical patients. *J Gen Intern Med* 1989; **4**: 23–30.

28 Renshaw DC. Coping with an impotent husband. *Illinois Med J* 1981; **159**: 29–33.

29 Basson R. Female sexual dysfunctions—the new models. *Br J Diabetes Vasc Dis* 2002; **2**: 267–70.

30 Tiefer L, Meleman A. Interviews of wives: a necessary adjunct in the evaluation of impotence. *Sex Disabil* 1983; **6**: 167–75.

31 EDIPC. *Erectile Dysfunction in Primary Care: Module 4.* Pfizer Ltd, 1998.

4

CHAPTER 5

Cardiovascular Disease and Sex

THE MYTH—SEX IS DANGEROUS

The myth that sex can be dangerous is perpetuated throughout history by media-hungry stories of public figures whose premature demise is seemingly linked to sexual activity. For example, in 1975 the former US vice president Nelson Rockefeller died at the age of 70 in the company of his 25-year-old-personal assistant Megan Marshack. According to *The Book of Lists*, Attila the Hun, the 5th century invader of Europe, also expired during the act. Other famous victims of coital death include Pope Leo VIII in 965 and former French president Felix Faure in 1899. Incidences such as these give rise to the incorrect assumption that normal sexual activity can be dangerous. Although clearly there have been cases of men expiring during the act of sexual intercourse, the odds of this happening stand at one sudden death per 1.51 million episodes of exertion [1]. In addition, studies have found that the majority of sexual activity-related sudden death episodes (around 75% of cases) usually involve an unfamiliar (and often much younger) partner, in an unfamiliar setting, and after excessive eating and alcohol consumption [2–4].

In terms of erectile dysfunction (ED), fear surrounding the safety of resuming or initiating sexual activity can in some instances play a large part in the development of sexual dysfunction, as well as affecting the overall effective management of the patient. For patients to resume normal sexual activity it is vital that their doctor or nurse is confident and able to reassure them that the risks involved are minimal.

THE REALITY—SEX IS LITERALLY A WALK IN THE PARK

The reality is that sex is just another form of exercise, and not necessarily a strenuous one at that. During sex the heart rate rises on average to 120–130 beats/min and systolic blood pressure rises to 150–180 mmHg. The duration of sex is normally between 5 and 15 min, with the peak effect taking place at

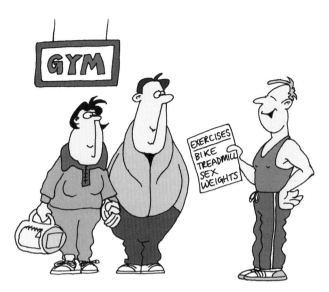

5

3–5 min (mean blood pressure at orgasm is 163/81) [5]. There is a small degree of cardiovascular risk associated with sexual activity among the general population, as there is with any mildly strenuous exercise, but this risk is not significantly increased in patients with stable cardiac disease. This risk decreases with regular physical exercise. Interestingly, although the peak heart rate during marital sex is on average 120 beats/min, during extramarital sex the heart rate can reach 180 beats/min!

As a gauge, the level of cardiac exertion for an activity can be expressed as the metabolic equivalent of the task (MET). One MET refers to the relative energy demand of oxygen usage in the resting state, which is approximately 3.5 mL oxygen/kg body weight per min [6]. Table 5.1 compares a number of daily activities in terms of their MET scores. To summarize, intercourse with an established partner equates to 2–3 METs with an upper range of 5–6 METs depending on how vigorous the activity is and the sexual positions adopted. This is equivalent to walking 1.5 km in 20 min, or climbing 20 stairs in 10 s. It is important to note that sex is no more strenuous to the heart than a number of other daily activities such as lifting and carrying objects or playing golf [6]. Anti-anginal therapy, such as β-blockers, may reduce the number of METs for a given degree of exercise by reducing the heart rate and blood pressure response to exertion.

Table 5.1 Metabolic equivalent of the task (MET) equivalents [6].

Daily activity	MET score rating
Sexual intercourse with an established partner	
Lower range ('normal')	2–3
Upper range (vigorous activity)	5–6
Lifting and carrying objects (9–20 kg)	4–5
Walking 1 mile in 20 min on the level	3–4
Golf	4–5
Gardening	3–5
DIY, wallpapering, etc.	4–5
Light housework, e.g. ironing, polishing	2–4
Heavy housework, e.g. making beds, scrubbing floors	3–6

DOES SEXUAL INTERCOURSE INCREASE THE RISK...
... of stroke?

Strokes occur most commonly at night and in the early morning, regardless of sexual activity. A coincidental occurrence of a stroke following sexual activity may result in survivors and partners assuming a strong relationship between the two. However, a recent study showed that sex does not significantly increase the risk of stroke and could even offer protection against fatal coronary events [7].

... of myocardial infarction?

Myocardial infarction (MI) can be triggered by exertion, anger and emotion, but in many cases the trigger is unknown. Patients are often wrongly fearful that sexual activity could precipitate an attack. One glance at the statistics should be enough to relieve these fears. During normal daily life the baseline risk of suffering an MI is only one chance in a million per hour for a healthy adult and 10 chances in a million per hour for a patient with pre-existing cardiovascular disease (CVD) (absolute risk) [8]. In the 2 h following sexual activity, the risk of MI increases 2.5-fold above baseline in the non-cardiovascular patient and about threefold in those with a history of prior MI. Therefore, the risk of triggering an MI in the cardiovascular patient following sex increases only a small amount to approximately 30 chances in a million per hour (compared with 10 chances in a million per hour during normal daily activity). In terms of percentages, this means that overall, sex is a likely contributor to MI in just under 1% of cases [8].

It is likely that the tension generated by sexual frustration can be more harmful than the excitement generated by sexual intercourse. A study by Bruhn in 1968 [9] found that MIs were associated with emotional drain and emotional stress—both of which can result from sexual frustration.

Relative risk of MI (95% CI) during 2 h after sexual activity [8]

All patients	2.5 (1.7–3.7)
Men	2.7 (1.8–4.0)
Women	1.3 (0.3–5.2)
Prior MI	2.9 (1.3–6.5)
Sedentary	3.0 (2.0–4.5)
Physically active	1.2 (0.4–3.7)

… in patients with diabetes?

ED is common in this group of patients and presentation with ED provides an opportunity to assess overall cardiovascular risk. Patients with Type 2 diabetes (approximately 80% of the overall diabetic population) require intensive management to improve their cardiovascular risk profile. Type 2 diabetic patients with no history of MI are at the same increased risk of developing an MI as non-diabetic patients who have had a previous MI [10]. It therefore follows that Type 2 diabetic risk factors should be treated just as aggressively as non-diabetic survivors of MI.

IDENTIFICATION AND MANAGEMENT OF ED IN THE CVD PATIENT
Broaching the subject of ED

Patients should be reassured that it is normal for men with CVD and diabetes to notice changes in their erectile function, as well as their sex drive. They should also be reassured that it is normal to be anxious about resuming sexual activity after illness. The assessment detailed in this chapter deals specifically with a cardiovascular patient; however, it should be borne in mind that as patients with diabetes (especially Type 2 diabetes) are at higher risk of cardiovascular complications such as hypertension and coronary heart disease, the following process also applies to assessment of ED in the diabetic patient. The majority of ED/CVD patients can be effectively assessed and treated within primary care.

Taking a history

Once the subject of erectile function has been raised and a potential problem identified, a full history of the erection problem should be taken to attempt to establish exactly what the cause of the ED could be. The sexual history should focus on:

> - Onset, frequency and severity of the ED
> - Situational or partner-specific problems
> - Presence of spontaneous early morning or nocturnal erections
> - History of perineal or back trauma or of abdominal or pelvic (including prostate) surgery

Even though the patient has CVD, it should not be automatically assumed that this must be the cause of the ED. It is important to eliminate other causes, such as a psychogenic cause. For example, clarifying whether the ED was of sudden or slow onset may help to identify whether the ED is mostly organic or psychogenic.

Factors to note during interview

> **Specific discussion points of the ED**
> - The problem as the patient sees it
> - Length of time since problem first occurred
> - Relationship (if any) between ED and the time, place or partner
> - Any loss of sex drive or dislike of sexual contact
> - Problems in the relationship
> - Stress factors as seen by the patient and their partner
> - Other anxiety, guilt or anger not expressed
> - Physical problems such as pain felt by either partner
>
> **General discussion points and background information**
> - Sexuality
> - Marital state
> - Expectations
> - Number of previous sexual partners
> - The current partner and duration of relationship
> - Number of children (if any) the patient has and where they live
> - Any obvious stress in the family
> - Any financial worries

Questionnaires may help to reduce the feelings of embarrassment that can arise when talking about sexual problems. The advantages and disadvantages of using questionnaires have already been discussed, but if this is an approach the primary healthcare team (PHCT) would like to use in its assessment, a number of questionnaires exist.

The ADAM questionnaire is one way to establish whether the patient may have hypogonadism-related erectile problems that need further investigation. The patient is asked 10 questions which have a yes or no answer. A positive response to questions 1 or 7, or any other three questions suggests the need for further investigation.

The ADAM questionnaire

1 Do you have decreasing libido?
2 Do you have a lack of energy?
3 Do you have a decrease in strength or endurance?
4 Have you lost height?
5 Have you decreased enjoyment of life?
6 Are you sad or grumpy?
7 Are your erections less strong?
8 Is it difficult to maintain your erection?
9 Are you falling asleep after dinner?
10 Has your work performance deteriorated recently?

Perhaps the most widely used and effective questionnaire for investigating a patient's erectile function is the International Index of Erectile Function (IIEF). A shortened adapted version of this questionnaire also exists in the form of the Sexual Health Inventory for Men (SHIM) (Table 5.2). With the use of SHIM 84.5% of patients reported an improvement in communication with their physician [11].

All patients with ED should also undergo a full medical assessment. This includes a medical history focusing on risk factors, such as cigarette smoking, hypertension, alcoholism, drug abuse, trauma and endocrine problems including hypothyroidism, low testosterone levels and hyperprolactinaemia. Finally, assessment of psychological history will help identify emotional issues such as interpersonal conflict, performance anxiety, depression or anxiety.

Physical assessment (Fig. 5.1)
Routine clinical examinations for ED should also be carried out in the cardiovascular patient experiencing problems with his erection, although laboratory tests should be kept to a minimum, limited to glucose, lipid profile and a morning serum testosterone, if the patient has a reduced libido [12]. A more detailed laboratory assessment should be carried out only if the PHCT feels it is indicated.

Table 5.2 Sexual Health Inventory for Men [12].

Patient's Name:_____   Date of Evaluation:_____

Sexual health is an important part of an individual's overall physical and emotional well-being. Erectile dysfunction, also known as impotence, is one type of a very common medical condition affecting sexual health. Fortunately, there are many different treatment options for erectile dysfunction. This questionnaire is designed to help you and your doctor identify if you may be experiencing erectile dysfunction. If you are, you may choose to discuss treatment options with your doctor.

Each question has several possible responses. Circle the number of the response that best describes you own situation. Please be sure that you select one and only one response for each question.

Over the past 6 months:
1 How do you rate your *confidence* that you could get and keep an erection?
Very low = 1
Low = 2
Moderate = 3
High = 4
Very high = 5

2 When you had erections with sexual stimulation, *how often* were your erections hard enough for penetration (entering your partner)?
No sexual activity = 0
Almost never or never = 1
A few times (much less than half the time) = 2
Sometimes (about half the time) = 3
Most times (much more than half the time) = 4
Almost always or always = 5

3 During sexual intercourse, *how often* were you able to maintain your erection after you had penetrated (entered) your partner?
Did not attempt intercourse = 0
Almost never or never = 1
A few times (much less than half the time) = 2
Sometimes (about half the time) = 3
Most times (much more than half the time) = 4
Almost always or always = 5

Table 5.2 (*Continued.*)

4 During sexual intercourse, *how difficult* was it to maintain your erection to completion of intercourse?
Did not attempt intercourse = 0
Extremely difficult = 1
Very difficult = 2
Difficult = 3
Slightly difficult = 4
Not difficult = 5

5 When you attempted sexual intercourse, *how often* was it satisfactory for you?
Did not attempt intercourse = 0
Almost never or never = 1
A few times (much less than half the time) = 2
Sometimes (about half the time) = 3
Most times (much more than half the time) = 4
Almost always or always = 5

Add the numbers corresponding to questions 1–5. If your score is 21 or less, you may be showing signs of erectile dysfunction and may want to speak with your doctor.
Score:_____

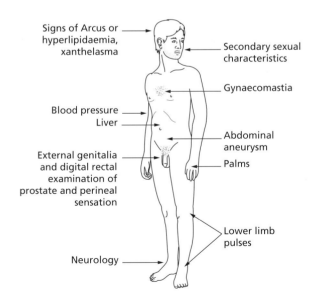

Fig. 5.1 Physical examination of men with erectile dysfunction.

Physical assessment
- Pressure
- Blood
- Femoral and peripheral pulses
- Femoral bruits (vascular abnormalities)
- A neurological examination exploring deep tendon reflexes, including bulbocavernosis reflex (assessed by noting an anal wink following a gentle squeeze of the glans penis)—if a neurological disease is suspected
- Sacral and perineal neurological exam (reduced sensation)
- Visual field defects (prolactinoma or pituitary mass)
- Breast exam (hyperprolactinaemia)
- Penile structure (Peyronie's disease)
- Testicular atrophy (testosterone deficiency)/asymmetry or masses of testes (hypogonadism)
- Rectal exam (allows for assessment of both the prostate and sphincter tone, abnormalities that are associated with autonomic dysfunction)
- Penile blood flow studies in special centres

RISK ANALYSIS FOR THE CARDIOVASCULAR PATIENT

Once the cause of the ED and a possible course of treatment have been identified, a risk assessment should be performed to determine whether a return to sexual activity is likely to trigger further cardiovascular events. Even with a normal exercise test or ECG, there are no guarantees that a person with pre-existing CVD is 100% risk-free. However, a thorough assessment can minimize this risk during which the PHCT should take into account the following points:

- Is there a fear of resuming sexual activity which is contributing to the ED?
- The greater the number of risk factors present, the greater the overall risk for the patient.
- When considering risk factors, the patient's previous sex drive, the effects of ageing, his partner's health and the patient's motivational state should all be taken into account.
- Establish the type of activities, frequency and level of physical exertion normally undertaken by the patient.
- Review the level of exertion of normal daily activities compared with the potential level of exertion in resuming sexual activity in terms of METs.

Risk factors for cardiovascular disease

- Hypertension
- Diabetes
- Smoking
- Hyperlipidaemia
- Chronic renal disease
- Age
- Ethnic background
- Gender
- Lifestyle, e.g. sedentary, alcohol
  and drug use

Associated clinical conditions:
angina
congestive heart failure
ischaemic heart disease
post-myocardial infarction
left ventricular failure
arrhythmias
left ventricular hypertrophy

EXERCISE TESTING TO EVALUATE SAFETY

The risk of a cardiac event is related to the patient's overall fitness and cardiovascular health. All ischaemic episodes during sexual intercourse are associated with an increased heart rate—if a patient experiences an ischaemic episode while on an exercise bicycle, they are also more likely to experience an ischaemic episode during sexual intercourse [13]. If the primary healthcare professional is in any doubt as to whether it is safe for their patient to resume or continue sexual activity, they should subject the patient to an exercise test. If a patient can achieve 5–6 METs (for 4 min) without significant ischaemia (> 2 mm ST-segment depression), arrhythmias or a fall in systolic blood pressure, the patient can be reassured that he is not at risk during normal sexual activity. Alternatively, the patient can be asked to walk 1 mile on the flat in 20 min. It is also useful if the partner observes the exercise testing, in terms of improving confidence of both the patient and his partner and hence reducing anxiety. If the patient does experience chest pain, extreme shortness of breath or irregular heartbeat during this activity, this may warrant further investigation into the patient's medical condition and its management before sexual activity can be pursued. Depending on the outcome of this investigation, the 'unfit' patient should commence a graduated exercise programme before having their exercise tolerance re-assessed at a later date using the same criteria.

A practical framework for assessing the potential level of cardiovascular risk following return to sexual activity has been devised (Table 5.3). Depending on the presenting condition, patients can be graded low, intermediate or high risk using these straightforward criteria.

Table 5.3 Management algorithm according to cardiovascular graded risk [14].

Grading of risk	Cardiovascular status upon presentat on	ED management recommendations for the primary care health professional
Low risk	• Controlled hypertension • Asymptomatic ≤ 3 risk factors for CAD—excluding age and gender • Mild valvular disease • Minimal/mild stable angina • Post successful revascularization • CHF (I)	• Manage within the primary care setting • Review treatment options with patient and his partner (where possible)
Intermediate risk	• Recent MI or CVA (i.e. within last 2–6 weeks) • LVD/CHF (II) • Murmur of unknown cause • Moderate stable angina • Heart transplant • Recurrent TIAs • Asymptomatic but >3 risk factors for CAD —excluding age and gender ⟷	• Specialized evaluation recommended (e.g. exercise test for angina, Echo for murmur) • Patient to be placed in high or low risk category, depending upon outcome of testing ⟶ • ED treatment can be initiated but exercise testing recommended to stratify risk
High risk	• Severe or unstable or refractory angina • Uncontrolled hypertension (SBP >180 mmHg) • CHF (III, IV) • Recent MI or CVA (i.e. within last 14 days) • High risk arrhythmias • Hypertrophic cardiomyopathy • Moderate/severe valve disease	• Refer for specialized cardiac evaluation and management • Treatment for ED to be deferred until cardiac condition established and/or specialist evaluation completed

CAD, coronary artery disease; MI, myocardial infarction; CVA, cerebral vascular accident; CHF, congestive heart failure; LVD, left ventricular dysfunction; SBP, systolic blood pressure; ED, erectile dysfunction; TIA, transient ischaemic attack.

New York Heart Association classification of congestive heart failure	
Class I	Patients with cardiac disease but with no limitation during ordinary physical activity
Class II	Slight limitations caused by cardiac disease. Activity such as walking causes dyspnoea
Class III	Marked limitation; symptoms are provoked easily, e.g. by walking on the flat
Class IV	Breathlessness at rest

Key considerations

• A myocardial infarction or stroke can be triggered by exertion, anger, emotion or, more rarely, sexual activity but in many cases the trigger is unknown. No guarantees can be given that a person with pre-existing cardiovascular disease is 100% risk-free from suffering further cardiovascular adverse events in the short or long term, even with a normal exercise test or ECG. However, the objective is to minimize this risk, through appropriate risk assessment.
• It is recognized that an exercise ECG is likely to have been conducted as part of the standard management process for many post-MI or angina patients, while under specialist care. If the MI is recent (less than 6 weeks) or if the healthcare professional is uncertain about symptom limitations, consideration should be given to further exercise testing

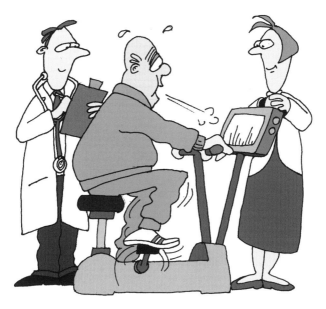

5

PATIENT PROFILES FROM THE THREE RISK CATEGORIES [15]
Low risk
The following types of cardiovascular conditions are regarded as low risk associated with sexual activity. Therefore, based on current knowledge, patients who fall in this category can usually be managed in primary care without the need for further investigations into their cardiac status and/or referral to a specialist.

> **Asymptomatic (less than three risk factors for coronary artery disease)**
> - Low risk for any significant cardiac complications from sexual activity or treatment of ED.
> - However, routine follow-up and monitoring of cardiovascular risk status important.
>
> **Controlled hypertension**
> - Regardless of the number or class of antihypertensive medications, these patients can be readily and safely managed with ED treatments.
> - Antihypertensive medication may be the cause of ED, although change in class or cessation of antihypertensive medication rarely results in restoration of erectile function.
> - Direct therapy for ED required.

Mild stable angina
- If angina previously evaluated and treated effectively, functional reserve is usually greater than that required by sexual activity.
- In borderline patient, medical management may preclude or prevent any symptoms during sexual activity (check with exercise stress test).
- Relative risk of acute non-fatal MI during sex in these patients no greater than in the patient without documented CVD.
- May need to modify angina drugs depending on sexual therapy regimen selected.

Post coronary artery bypass graft (CABG) or percutaneous coronary intervention (angioplasty, stenting, etc.)
- Risk is dependent on adequacy of the revascularization.
- Exercise stress testing can assess the extent and severity of residual ischaemia.
- If adequate revascularization and no significant residual ischaemia, patient is low risk.

Past MI (more than 6–8 weeks post-MI)
- Post-MI sexual activity is safe for the large majority of patients following 6–8-week recovery period.
- Advise patient to start with low key kisses and caresses, and as health and confidence grow, resume normal sexual activities.
- If post-MI stress test is satisfactory, recovery period may be reduced to 3–4 weeks in selected patients.
- Completion of exercise test of 4–5 METs beforehand will determine risk and provide reassurance.
- Exercise training post-MI will improve cardiovascular efficiency and reduce myocardial oxygen consumption during sexual activity [8].
- Cardiac rehabilitation exercise programmes reduce reported coital symptoms and reduce coital heart rates.

Mild mitral valvular disease
- Patient not at greatly increased risk for coition-induced cardiac events.
- Also true of select cases of aortic stenosis.
- Male patients can safely employ oral, intraurethral or injectable medications without need for antibiotic prophylaxis.

Mild congestive heart failure (Class I)
- Defined as cardiac disease that allows ordinary physical activity without symptoms.
- No increased risk of coition-induced cardiac events.

Other cardiovascular conditions
- Atrial fibrillation with controlled ventricular response.

- Mitral valve prolapse.
- Pericarditis.
- Risk of sexual activity not really known in these patients.
- If unsure, further cardiac tests should be conducted.

Intermediate risk

Patients who are classified as being at intermediate risk should not resume sexual activity or undergo treatment for ED until their cardiac status has been re-evaluated and they have been restratified into either the high-risk or low-risk category. A consultation with a cardiologist may be useful in some cases to help determine the relative safety of sexual activity for the individual.

Asymptomatic with more than three cardiovascular risk factors
- Should consider cardiovascular assessment, for example, exercise stress test.
- Sedentary lifestyle is an important risk factor—would justify a fitness programme and possibly an exercise stress test.

Moderate, stable angina
- Ischaemia is usually reproducible in the stable angina patient for a given exercise-induced heart rate and systolic blood pressure increase.
- Exercise test would further predict risk of acute cardiac events among patients with coronary artery disease.

History of MI (between 2 and 4 weeks post-MI)
- May be at slightly higher risk of ischaemia and re-infarction during sexual intercourse, as well as malignant arrhythmia.
- Risk may be assessed by exercise stress testing.

Left ventricular dysfunction/congestive heart failure (Class II)
- Slight limitations caused by cardiac disease, with activities such as walking causing dyspnoea.
- Moderate risk for exacerbation with sexual activity.
- Cardiovascular assessment, rehabilitation and treatment may facilitate re-classification to a low-risk category.

Non-cardiac sequelae of atherosclerotic disease
- Patients with clinically evident peripheral arterial disease, history of stroke or transient ischaemic attacks are at higher risk of MI.
- Patients should be considered for cardiovascular evaluation.

5

High risk

High-risk patients are defined as those whose cardiac condition is sufficiently severe that sexual activity could be a risk. ED in these patients should not be managed in primary care, they should be referred for further cardiac assessment by a specialist. Sexual activity should be deferred until either the condition has stabilized with treatment or a cardiologist has decided that sexual activity may safely be resumed.

Unstable, refractory angina
- Angina that is new onset, severe, accelerated, refractory or occurs at rest.
- Patients who have functional reserve that is exceeded by mild physical activity, typically including intercourse.
- These patients have potentially higher risk of MI during exercise or sexual intercourse.

Uncontrolled hypertension
- Untreated, poorly controlled, accelerated or malignant hypertension.
- These patients are at risk of acute cardiac and vascular events, including stroke.

Congestive heart failure (Class III/IV)
- Defined as breathless at rest (IV).
- Marked limitation with symptoms provoked easily (e.g. walking on flat) (III).
- Sexual activity may trigger cardiac decompensation in some patients.

Recent MI (less than 2 weeks)
- May be at risk for coition-induced reinfarction, cardiac rupture or perhaps coition-induced arrhythmias [13].
- Period of maximum risk is within 2 weeks of MI.
- Patient should be advised to generally rest and under no circumstances resume sexual activity.

High-risk arrhythmias
- Malignant arrhythmias during sexual activity are a rare cause of sudden death.
- Patient with ventricular arrhythmia, particularly if induced by exercise or coition, is at high risk.
- Holter monitoring during sexual activity may be of value in selected cases.
- Patients with implanted defibrillators or pacemakers not at any greater risk.

Hypertrophic obstructive cardiomyopathy
- Relatively rare, but associated with syncope and sudden death during or after exercise.
- Vasodilators may increase the intraventricular gradient and should be specifically avoided in these patients.

- Exercise stress testing and ECG should guide management with regard to effort-induced symptoms or arrhythmias.

Moderate to severe valve disease (especially aortic stenosis)
- Significant aortic stenosis associated with sudden death.
- Vasoactive drugs should be used with caution in these patients as may not tolerate systemic vasodilation, with resultant decrease in perfusion pressure in the coronary and cerebrovascular circulation.

SUMMARY OF RISK ASSESSMENT (Fig. 5.2)

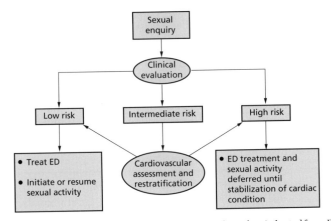

Fig. 5.2 Sexual activity and cardiac risk—a simplified algorithm (adapted from Debusk *et al.* (2000) [15]).

TREATMENT OPTIONS FOR ED IN THE CVD PATIENT [14]
To minimize the risk of a cardiac event associated with the patient resuming sexual activity, management of ED in patients with CVD should always be secondary to stabilizing their cardiovascular status and optimizing their drug therapy for their cardiovascular symptoms.

All currently licensed ED treatments are suitable for managing ED in the cardiovascular patient, provided the manufacturer's instructions are adhered to. With two exceptions, advantages and disadvantages of each treatment option are the same for the cardiovascular patient as for any other, and do not increase the overall cardiovascular risk in patients with diagnosed CVD, provided they are used correctly.

These exceptions are:

> - Patients on Warfarin—may experience increased risk of bruising with injections, urethral bleeding with intraurethral alprostadil and haematoma with the vacuum device.
> - Patients on nitrate therapy—sildenafil is contraindicated and apomorphine is cautioned.

There is no evidence that any form of ED therapy increases cardiac risk, assuming all instructions are followed. Sexual intercourse is no more stressful to the heart than many other normal daily activities.

The multicentre Investigation of Limitation of Infarct Size Study [16] found that less than 50% of patients reported a triggering activity for their MI, so some events will occur simply coincidentally following commencement of ED therapy, particularly in an age group at risk of ischaemic heart disease. The most extensive published data reviewing efficacy and safety of ED treatments in cardiovascular patients relate to sildenafil.

Risk of adverse events/MI with sildenafil citrate

The first phase of prescription event monitoring of cardiovascular events in 5600 sildenafil users concluded that there is no evidence for a higher incidence of fatal MI or ischaemic heart disease among men taking sildenafil [17]. Other studies have found:

> - No evidence of adverse events in men with severe CAD [18].
> - Sildenafil is well tolerated and does not change the onset, extent or severity of ischaemia in men with coronary artery disease [19,20].
> - No evidence to support sildenafil as a cause of serious cardiac events [21].

GENERAL EFFICACY IN CARDIOVASCULAR PATIENT

In terms of efficacy in this specific group of patients, once again, the only published subgroup data on ED treatments in cardiovascular patients relate to sildenafil. Twenty-one randomized placebo controlled trials have demonstrated that sildenafil improves erectile function and improves intercourse rates, including in those with diabetes and CVD, by 70–90% compared with 10–30% for those patients on placebo [22].

SPECIAL CONSIDERATIONS FOR THE DIABETIC PATIENT

Maintaining metabolic control in diabetic patients is crucial and it is extremely important that pharmacological treatments for ED do not adversely affect glucose or lipid homeostasis. Treatments must not interact with other medications that diabetic men frequently require, e.g. insulin, oral antidiabetic, antihypertensive or lipid-lowering drugs. There is no indication that sildenafil affects blood glucose levels in diabetic patients or that it impairs metabolic control [23]. Therefore sildenafil is highly suitable for administration to diabetic patients.

The data for efficacy of apomorphine in diabetic patients are less strong—this may be because apomorphine is a centrally acting agent and therefore may not be as effective in men with severe corpora cavernosal endothelial cell dysfunction, as seen in those patients with diabetes.

ORAL THERAPY AND NITRATES

Sildenafil is absolutely contraindicated in patients taking nitrate therapy or nitric oxide donors, whether their treatment is given regularly or intermittently.

If the cardiovascular patient is taking nitrates, there are two options in order for the patient to be considered safe to resume sexual activity:

- Suggest an alternative form of ED therapy—the patient and partner should be fully counselled regarding the rationale for this.
- Transfer the patient to an alternative anti-ischaemic therapy such as a β-blocker or calcium channel blocker and discontinue nitrate therapy completely. This is possible in most angina patients because nitrates are a symptomatic treatment and do not have prognostic significance. However, if the patient's condition is complex the opinion of a cardiologist should be sought.

Although the mechanism of action of Uprima is different from that of sildenafil, and it has been found to be well tolerated in patients who are also taking nitrates (incidence of treatment-related side-effects (14.1%) is similar to those not taking Uprima with nitrates (16.9%)), caution is still advised in administrating Uprima concurrently with nitrates [24].

GETTING FIT FOR SEX

If ever there was a reason to start a fitness programme, this is it. Although the absolute risk of MI is low, regular physical activity further reduces the risk of triggering an MI by sexual activity.

Case crossover study of 699 MI patients (sexually active, 560; age 45–70 (mean 59) years; women, 50%) [25]

Risk of MI (95%CI) during 1 h after sexual activity (Sweden):	
All patients	2.1 (0.7–6.5)
Sedentary	4.4 (1.5–12.9)
Physically active	0.7 (0.1–5.1)

As an added incentive, it has been found that men who maintain a moderate level of physical activity level of at least 200 kcal/day have a lower risk of ED [26], and it is never too late to increase physical activity and reap the benefits. The same study found that the risk of ED was significantly reduced among men who were sedentary at baseline and became physically active during the course of the study [26].

Exercise can also lower the risk of stroke. Men who are physically fit and maintain a regular aerobic exercise programme are less likely to suffer a stroke than their sedentary peers. This is largely because exercise lowers the risk of hypertension, obesity and diabetes. Men who are able to exercise for long periods are less likely to have a stroke—and this relationship exists regardless of weight, smoking, alcohol or parent's history of heart disease, hypertension and diabetes. The most aerobically fit are deemed 68% less likely to have a stroke than their more unfit peers. The moderately fit are 63% less likely to have a stroke [27].

FOLLOW-UP OF ED/CVD PATIENTS

It is very important that the cardiovascular/diabetic patient is reviewed regularly to assess the patient's cardiovascular status and response to the ED therapy. To maximize positive outcomes from initiation of ED therapy, the following points should be taken into consideration:

- Patients often expect instant success with their treatment.
- Many patients do not give therapy an adequate chance simply through misunderstanding or not following instructions, e.g. not realizing that sexual stimulation is required for some treatments.
- In view of the impact of further erectile failure on the patient's self-esteem, the patient should be advised that treatment may be successful only after several trials and some erectile failure.
- A follow-up appointment shortly after the initial assessment and prescription of therapy can improve compliance through managing the patient and partner's expectations of treatment and increase confidence with therapy.
- The impact of the resumption of sexual activity and the concurrent increased level of exertion on the patient's cardiovascular status should be monitored.
- The patient should report any episodes of pain during sexual activity so that any treatment for angina can be reviewed and modified.
- Once the patient is stable on their ED treatment, patient follow-up and reassessment at regular intervals (e.g. every 6 months) is recommended.
- After a certain period of time it should be discussed whether the patient has had any return of spontaneous erections.

KEY POINTS

- Sex is no more stressful to the heart than a round of golf or walking 1 mile in 20 min.
- Cardiac risk assessment should be included in the initial evaluation of all cardiovascular (and diabetic) patients.
- The majority of patients assessed to be at low or intermediate cardiac risk can be effectively managed in primary care.
- An exercise test can help determine whether it is safe for the patient to resume sexual activity.
- There is no evidence that currently licensed treatments for ED add to the overall cardiovascular risk in patients with or without diagnosed CVD.

REFERENCES

1 Albert CM, Mittleman MA, Chase CU *et al.* Triggering of sudden death from cardiac causes by vigorous exertion. *N Engl J Med* 2000; **343**: 1355–61.

2 Parzellar M, Raschka C, Bratzke H. Sudden cardiovascular death in correlation with sexual activity—results of a medicolegal postmortem study from 1972–1998. *Eur Heart J* 2001; **22**: 610–1.

3 Ueno M. The so-called coition death. *Jpn J Legal Med* 1963; **127**: 333–40.

4 Krauland W. Unerwarteter Tod—Herzinfarkt und Sexualitat aus der Sicht des Rechtsmediziners. *Sexualmedizin* 1976; **10** (S): 20–3.

5 Nemeo *et al. Am Heart J* 1976; **92**: 274.

6 Wilson PK, Farday PS, Froelicher V, eds. *Cardiac Rehabilitation: Adult Fitness and Exercise Testing*. Philadelphia: Lea & Fabiger, 1981.

7 Ebrahim S, May M, Schlomo BY *et al.* Sexual intercourse and risk of ischaemic stoke and coronary heart disease: the Caerphilly study. *J Epidemiol Community Health* 2002; **56**: 99–102.

8 Müller JE, Mittleman A, Maclure M, Sherwood JB, Tofler GH. Determinants of Myocardial Infarction Onset Study Investigators. Triggering myocardial infarction by sexual activity. Low absolute risk and prevention by regular physical exertion. *JAMA* 1996; **275**: 1405–9.

9 Bruhn JGMC, Crady K, DuPlessis AL. Evidence of 'emotional drain' preceding death from myocardial infarction. *Psychiat Dig* 1968; **29**: 34–40.

10 Haffner SM, Lehto S, Ronnemaa T. Mortality from coronary heart disease in subjects with type 2 diabetes and in nondiabetic subjects with and without prior myocardial infarction. *N Engl J Med* 1998; **333**: 229–34.

11 Stecher VJ, Siegel R. Assessment of communication level between physicians and patients following use of the sexual health inventory for men, a diagnostic tool for erectile dysfunction. 1999.

12 Levine LA, Kloner AR. Importance of asking questions about erectile dysfunction. *Am J Cardiol* 2000; **86**: 1210–3.

5

13 Drory Y, Shapira I, Fisman EZ, Pines A. Myocardial ischemia during sexual activity in patients with coronary artery disease. *Am J Cardiol* 1995; **15**: 1321–2.

14 Jackson G, Betteridge J, Dean J *et al.* A systematic approach to erectile dysfunction in the cardiovascular patient: a consensus statement. *Int J Clin Pract* 1999; **53**: 445–51.

15 Debusk R, Drory Y, Goldstein I *et al.* Management of sexual dysfunction in patients with cardiovascular disease: recommendations of the Princeton Consensus panel. *Am J Cardiol* 2000; **86**: 62F–68F.

16 Tofler GH, Stone PH, Maclure M *et al.* Analysis of possible triggers of acute myocardial infarction (the MILIS study). *Am J Cardiol* 1990; **66**: 22–7.

17 Shakir SAW, Wilton LV, Boshier A, Layton D, Heeley E. Cardiovascular events in users of sildenafil: results from first phase of prescription event monitoring in England. *BMJ* 2001; **322**: 651–2.

18 Herrmann HC, Chang G, Klugherz BD, Mahoney PD. Hemodynamic effects of sildenafil in men with severe coronary artery disease. *N Engl J Med* 2000; **342**: 1622–6.

19 Patrizi R, Leonardo F, Pelliccia F *et al.* Effect of sildenafil citrate upon myocardial ischemia in patients with chronic stable angina in therapy with beta-blockers. *Ital Heart J* 2001; **2**: 841–4.

20 Arruda-Olson AM, Mahoney DW, Nehra A, Leckel M, Pellikka PA. Cardiovascular effects of sildenafil during exercise in men with known or probable coronary artery disease: a randomized crossover trial. *JAMA* 2002; **287**: 719–25.

21 Sadovsky R, Miller T, Moskowitz M, Hackett G. Three-year update of sildenafil citrate (Viagra®) efficacy and safety. *Int J Clin Pract* 2001; **55**: 115–28.

22 Osterloh I. Update on the efficacy and safety of Viagra. In: *VII International Symposium of Andrology*, Palma, Mallorca, 2000.

23 Price DE, Boolell M, Gepi-Attee S *et al.* Study of a novel oral treatment for erectile dysfunction in diabetic men. *Diabet Med* 1998; **15**: 821–5.

24 Heaton J. *EAU*, Birmingham, 2002.

25 Moller J, Ahlbom A, Hulting J *et al.* Sexual activity as a trigger of myocardial infarction. A case-crossover analysis in the Stockholm Heart Epidemiology Programme (SHEEP). *Heart* 2001; **86**: 387–90.

26 Johannes CB, Araujo A, Feldman HA *et al.* Incidence of erectile dysfunction (ED) in ageing men: longitudinal results from Massachusetts Male Ageing Study (MMAS). *Int J Impot Res* 1998; **10**: S55.

27 Lee CD, Blair SN. Cardiorespiratory fitness and stroke mortality in men. *Med Sci Sports Exerc* 2002; **34**: 592–5.

CHAPTER 6

Well Man and Erectile Dysfunction Clinics in General Practice

Throughout the centuries, expectations in society have led to men being perceived as being the 'strong' gender. Consequently, men have a very functional view of their bodies and 'expect' it to continue working successfully, regardless of the task set for it. Men generally have no reason to pay attention to their bodies until an external factor becomes involved—for example, alcohol consumption, physical exertion or an accident.

However, women are used to constant change taking place within their bodies throughout their life—from the onset of menstruation, to pregnancy, giving birth, and eventually menopause. Men do begin to experience physical changes to their bodies as they enter middle age, but it is only when their bodies start to malfunction that men begin to realize that their health is actually vulnerable. Even with this realization, men remain generally reluctant to visit

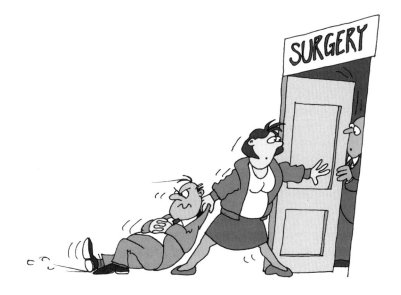

the doctor, for fear of being labelled a hypochondriac or for 'making a fuss' about nothing.

ATTENDING THE SURGERY—MEN VS. WOMEN

Most women are comfortable discussing their health and their health symptoms with their friends, and so have fewer concerns about discussing the same issues with a doctor or nurse. However, health is rarely a topic of conversation amongst men, and especially not when the topic concerns a potentially embarrassing condition that may reflect badly on their image and sense of masculinity, such as problems of a sexual nature or involving the sexual organs. Consequently, men find it more difficult to discuss certain health topics with their doctor or nurse than do women and may also feel that they lack the necessary vocabulary to discuss their symptoms.

Women tend to have a closer relationship with the healthcare system than men, due mainly to their having much more cause to visit the doctor's surgery throughout their lives than men, whether it be due to requiring prescribed contraceptives, health screening, pregnancy, childbirth or the care of young children. There are very few services provided that address men's health specifically, although this may change in the future.

MAKING THE SURGERY 'MALE-FRIENDLY'

Men would be much more likely to attend the doctor's surgery if services were made 'male-friendly'. There is compelling evidence that more men would present for treatment if there were more points of access for information and treatment about sexual problems, including telephone services, websites and walk-in clinics, as well as the traditional surgery appointment. The aim must be to remove the stigma attached to men visiting their doctor and instead ensure that this becomes simply part of a normal health routine.

One approach to making services 'male-friendly' is to give men the opportunity to attend the surgery during hours which fit in with their working lifestyle, e.g. in the evenings or during lunch time. Regular surgery hours mean that men usually have to negotiate with employers to attend an appointment. Men may fear that this process will raise doubts with their employer over their ability to perform their role at work, as well as eating into their working day. It has been found that initiatives where health services actually seek out men, e.g. work-based clinics, tend to be more successful than those relying on men to go to a health centre. If opening hours and locations of services were made more accessible to men, and advertised effectively, it is likely that more men would utilize services. Outreach clinics in community settings have attracted large numbers of men because they offer a service that meets the needs of men, including information, at a time and place that is convenient to those men who need help.

THE WELL MAN CLINIC

A Well Man clinic can be an effective way of encouraging men into the surgery, and organizing health services for men can have positive effects on the practice as a whole. The more regularly men present to their doctor, the earlier diseases can be identified and treatment initiated. The financial implications of this earlier identification and treatment are significant. The earlier diseases are identified and treated, the fewer days are lost to sickness in the workplace and the shorter and less frequent the stays in hospital. Targets set out in National Frameworks (and the *Health of the Nation*) are more likely to be met.

Benefits of developing a Well Man clinic

- Quality of care
- Health promotion payments
- Healthier patients
- Team building
- Audit
- Patient demand
- *Health of the Nation* targets
- Proven clinical effectiveness
- More effective use of resources
- Greater utilization of data collected
- Sensitive to local healthcare need
- Optimized purchasing decisions

6

ESSENTIAL STEPS TO DEVELOPING AN EFFICIENT WELL MAN CLINIC

1. Decide who will provide medical care

The present-day healthcare system requires a number of different skills. Teamwork is the key to efficient health promotion and prevention of illness in a Well Man clinic. The clinic can be included in the working week of 37.5 h and at least two medically qualified staff should be present (at least one nurse and one doctor). Typically a team includes the following members:

Practice nurse or health visitor

Men should present to the nurse for the initial health screening, and only be referred to the GP if the outcome of the initial investigations suggests that medical intervention is needed. Nurses should include asking about erectile function as part of their general Well Man screening.

Doctor

Although patients will present to the nurse initially, a doctor should be on hand to deal with any referrals, questions or further investigations that arise.

Team leader—financial and medical responsibility

Usually takes the lead with regard to decisions regarding medical input and managing finances. This is usually the doctor.

Receptionist

Co-ordinator for patient enquiries, appointments and referrals. Also collects information and compiles reports for audit purposes.

2. Develop effective teamwork

It is vital to have shared goals and understanding of each others' roles. One way of developing effective procedures and interpersonal relationships is to use a SWOT analysis: the group meets and discusses and agrees the current strengths (S), weaknesses (W), opportunities (O) and threats (T) in setting up a Well Man clinic. Examples of factors relevant to each area are as follows:

SWOT analysis in the development of a Well Man clinic [1]

Strengths	Opportunities
Committed team	Learning
Clear protocol	Disease prevention
Sound knowledge base	Healthier, happier patients
Convenient appointment times	Financial support
Health authority support	Increased quality of care
Health promotion committee approval	New practice partner enthusiastic
Patients' appreciation	Practice staff enthusiastic
Variety of work	
Weaknesses	**Threats**
Premises in poor repair	Lack of motivation
Inadequate space	Falling practice size
Nurse needs computer terminal	Staff member leaving
None of the present team has experience in sexual health	Future funding uncertain
	Political change in the NHS
Staff already have time pressures	Time pressures
Generates more work	Financial shortage
Time not convenient	Cost of training

Factors affecting the establishment of a successful Well Man clinic team [2]

Qualities of effective leadership
1 Inspires trust
2 Selects good staff
3 Has infectious enthusiasm
4 Is a good listener
5 Runs effective meetings
6 Good presenter
7 Accepts responsibility
8 Can tolerate uncertainties
9 Responds positively to conflict and failure
10 Has a good sense of humour
11 Maintains good morale

Factors helpful to team morale
1 Small organization that communicates well
2 High quality and level of training of staff
3 High motivation and dedication
4 Clear sense of direction and goals shared by all
5 Organizational stability and low staff turnover
6 Sensitive to patients' needs
7 Quality assurance with results shared with all concerned
8 Regular reports of progress towards goals and targets
9 An open style of organization and leadership
10 Adaptability to change
11 Ability to contain conflict where used constructively

How to measure the quality of team work
1 The views and judgement of people concerned, such as patients, staff, authorities, other professional teams, using appropriate criteria
2 The innovativeness of the team
3 Team vision and shared objectives
4 Participative safety, implying that the team is seen by members as supportive and that information is safe within the team
5 Commitment to excellence and a shared concern for quality of the team and individual performance
6 Audit activity
7 Re-audit to assess change

6

3. Set goals for men's health

The team must have a shared understanding of men's health. This can be initiated by a brainstorm meeting to discuss key areas of men's health, raise awareness of the diseases from which men suffer and to construct a systematic, protocolled approach to selective disease groups and/or health screening. The team must also establish the overall aims of the clinic:

- Provide accurate and thorough current health information to men
- Search systematically for disease where early detection is important
- Monitor and adjust for chronic conditions and monitor borderline abnormalities

4. Arrange meeting to discuss practicalities

The following practicalities need to be addressed in order to ensure the successful execution of a Well Man clinic [1]:

1 Agree the partner or colleague for the project
2 Define practice priorities in terms of which services need to be provided and which disease areas are important
3 Literature search and future meeting to present results of this
4 Establish everyone's responsibilities—who will do what, where and when
5 Agree timing of clinics and provisional start date
6 Define patient target group, e.g. men aged 45–70
7 Estimate numbers of patients attending the clinic
8 Define length of appointments
9 Clarify how staff can get access to a doctor if questions arise during consultation or prescriptions needed
10 Inform patients about the clinic
   - practice notice board
   - practice leaflet
   - opportunities during consultation
   - computer searches
   - disease indexes
   - local newspaper publicity
11 Arrangements for appointments and recall, systematic or opportunistic; make a decision regarding whether non-attenders will be reappointed
12 Cultural/language implications/specific approach to men with learning difficulties?/disabled or house bound
13 Get approval from the Health Promotion Committee
14 Develop an audit trail

5. Devise a protocol

The clinic can function effectively only if there is a clear understanding of the agreed procedures and guidelines. It needs to be established what information is to be recorded and where. Involving all members of the team in this process is an important factor in keeping the clinic focused and the staff interested and motivated, as well as facilitating audit and report. Protocol trends need to be promptly recognized, allowing the staff to attach value to what they are doing. With each attendance, the minimum data required of each patient should be recorded, and at regular defined intervals. Data from all the patients seen in the clinic should be collated by a named individual in order to complete an audit.

Sample protocol for a Well Man clinic [1] (can be downloaded from the website www.edvasculardisease.com)

Personal data
Name
Date of birth
Address
Occupation
Marital status
Employment situation
Smoking status
Average alcohol consumption
Sexual orientation (if relevant)
Enquire about skin health and discuss avoidance of sunburn

Health problems
Current and significant past

Therapy history
Current medication
Prescription and self-medication

Family history
- Heart disease
- Prostate cancer
- Other forms of cancer
- High blood pressure
- Hypothyroidism
- Gout
- Stroke
- Diabetes
- Epilepsy

Cholesterol
- Ever tested?
- Needs testing?

Stress

Enquire about level of stress and consider the use of a rating scale. Reinforce advice regarding safe limits of alcohol.

Depression

Enquire about depression and consider use of a rating scale.

Accidents

Eyesight check, take care with prescribed drugs when driving; don't drink and drive; all drugs at home to be kept under lock and key.

Sexual health

Discuss safe sex methods and precautions against sexually transmitted diseases; advise use of condoms and reduction of numbers of sexual partners.

Exercise history

How much and how often, daily exercise where possible, but at least 20 min three times a week. Steps to ensure safe exercise:

- Wear suitable footwear, preferably with ankle support and designed for walking or jogging.
- Consider the use of shock-absorbing inserts if there is arthritis pain in knees or hips.
- Drink plenty of water before and after exercise.
- Wear clothing that allows ease of movement and evaporation of water.
- Avoid exercising outdoors in very warm or very cold weather.
- Stop exercising immediately if the following symptoms occur: chest pain, shortness of breath, dizziness, light-headedness or palpitations.
- Do not exercise if suffering from any infectious condition, such as a cold or influenza.
- Consider supervised training in a gymnasium.
- Exercise with a partner if possible.

Prostate health

Ask the following questions:

- Are you bothered by urinary function?
- Do you get up at night to pass water?
- Have you noticed a deterioration in your urinary stream?

An affirmative answer should lead to the use of the International Prostate Symptom Score and Quality of Life Assessment.

Testicular health

Offer a leaflet on self-examination.

Osteoporosis risk
Provide check-lists for risk factors for osteoporosis in men and consider use of DXA scan to evaluate if positive.

Risk factors:

- Previous fracture
- Alcohol excess
- Intestinal disease
- Thyroid disease
- Low calcium intake
- Anticonvulsant therapy

- Hypogonadism
- Heavy smoking
- Gastric surgery
- Hypercalciuria
- Family history of fractures caused by osteoporosis

- Anorexia nervosa
- Steroid use
- COPD
- Coeliac disease
- Ankylosing spondylitis

Examination
- Height/weight: calculate and explain the BMI.
- Measure waist circumference: larger waist circumference identifies people at increased cardiovascular risk.
- Blood pressure: < 140/85 mmHg, reassure and recommend a further check, not longer than 5 years; 140/85–150/90 mmHg, recommend annual review; unless patient is diabetic or has other cardiovascular risk factors ≥150/90 mmHg, repeat three times over the next 4 weeks and then review with the GP.
- Rectal examination where appropriate.

Investigations
- Urinalysis: dipstick test for blood, glucose and protein; if abnormal, send MSU to laboratory; ensure the patient has instructions for collection of MSU and refer patient to GP for advice.
- Peak expiratory flow rate.
- Consider use of vitalograph if early COPD suspected.

Blood tests
- Blood cholesterol: where indicated according to other cardiovascular risk factors.
- HIV and PSA test should not be requested without suitable pretest counselling.

Review all data collected
Give advice and appropriate leaflets on smoking, diet and weight control, exercise, lifestyle, avoidance of sunburn, sexual health, family history of coronary heart disease, any previous cardiovascular events, prostate health, testicular health and bone health.

Immunizations
Ensure the patient is fully immunized according to approved guidelines.

6

Follow-up

If no problems detected, offer repeat appointment in 5 years; if any significant abnormality detected, refer to doctor.

Audit

Every 6 months audit data will be reviewed, numbers seen and non-attenders, problems detected, outcomes, consider patient satisfaction survey.

Complaints

Referral to practice-based complaints procedure at earliest opportunity.

Current concerns

Any questions about health that are worrying the patient at this time.

Erectile dysfunction

Patients should be routinely asked about their erectile function—for example:
- Have you noticed any difficulty obtaining or maintaining your erections?

Many primary-care practitioners are considering the advisability of setting up an in-house service for erectile dysfunction.

Patients with a history of heart disease

A focused history and examination in these patients is important because they are at high absolute risk for further problems with a four- to eightfold increased risk of recurrence; there is also good evidence of benefit, and risk management and treatment are cost effective. This is a special group that needs an additional protocol:

1 History of cardiac event
2 Date of admission to hospital
3 What diagnosis was made?
4 Details of current medication
5 Is the patient compliant with medication?
6 Is blood pressure controlled?
7 Is the patient currently smoking?
8 Hospital follow-up arrangements
9 What tests have been performed:
  - Cholesterol
  - Has diabetes been excluded?
  - ECG
  - Exercise treadmill test
  - Echocardiogram
10 Are there any current complaints:

- Chest pain
- Palpitations
- Shortness of breath
- Cough
- Ankle swelling
- Orthopnoea
- Paroxysmal nocturnal dyspnoea

Check patient is on aspirin
Aspirin should be in routine use unless there is a contraindication.

ACE inhibitor indicated
Consider the use of ACE inhibition if the patient has a past history of cardiac failure, hypertension, diabetes or microalbuminuria.

Investigations
- BMI
- Blood pressure
- Blood lipids
- Blood sugar
- Urinalysis
- Echocardiogram
- ECG

Review of history and examination
Be prepared to give advice with appropriate supportive literature on cardiac symptoms, smoking, alcohol, exercise, cardiac rehabilitation programme, diet and obesity, medication, reinforce importance of regular follow-up. Are the blood lipids in the target area? Is the patient on aspirin? Is an ACE inhibitor indicated? Was the patient prescribed a β-blocker and has it been continued? Is there any indication for the use of anticoagulation: for example, has the patient ever been, or is he currently, in atrial fibrillation?

Key to abbreviations: ACE, angiotensin-converting enzyme; BMI, body mass index; COPD, chronic obstructive pulmonary disease; DEXA, dual energy X-ray absorptiometry; ECG, electrocardiogram; HIV, human immunodeficiency virus; MSU, midstream urine; PSA, prostate-specific antigen.

Ongoing education

It is very important in terms of practising evidence-based medicine and running the clinic effectively, that all members of the team are updated regularly on all aspects of men's health. Educational meetings should be held within the practice, literature searches should be regularly undertaken and relevant key papers and articles on men's health circulated to all team members to meet their educational needs. Joint attendance at postgraduate meetings also fosters a team approach.

6. Include an ED service within the Well Man clinic

Given men's natural reticence to discuss sexual problems (among those experiencing erectile dysfunction (ED), 40% of diabetics and 50% of the control had never discussed their problem [3]), a Well Man clinic is a particularly appropriate environment in which to raise the subject of ED with patients (along with routine diabetic and cardiovascular clinics). It should be borne in mind that it is not uncommon for there to be a considerable delay between the onset of the sexual problem and presentation at the clinic, ranging from a few weeks to over 40 years [4]. Therefore, a service to identify and manage men with ED should be an integral part of any Well Man clinic.

Requirements for providing a primary care ED service
Clinical knowledge and skill requirements
In order to identify and manage ED effectively the PHCT should have knowledge of:

- Basic sexual physiology and psychology
- Chronic disease
- Drugs and therapeutics

And skills in:
- Consultation
- Counselling
- Physical examination
- Practice management

In addition, the PHCT should have knowledge of:
- Physiology and pathophysiology of erection
- Psychological and physical treatments for ED
- Management strategies (including referral and follow-up options)

Time for ED consultation
It is prudent to allow 20–30 min for an initial consultation, to include history-taking and examination. Further time, perhaps 10–15 min, should be allowed

for explanation and discussion of treatment. If patients need tuition in the use of a given treatment, further time will be required for this.

Liaison with local secondary care providers
The PHCT should explore pre-existing services that may already be available locally. These can include a secondary care-based psychosexual therapy service, an ED clinic or services provided by voluntary agencies such as RELATE. It is worth contacting these services to establish exactly what they provide and also to find out their qualifications and experience. It is useful to build up a good relationship with these services—knowledge of each other's interests and clinic procedures should result in more efficient and effective patient care in terms of:

- More effective referral procedures
- Appropriate use of follow-up in both primary and secondary care
- Availability of advice and support for ED management
- Availability of emergency assistance in the management of priapism
- Opportunities for collaboration and shared learning

ED clinics in secondary care
This is a clinic specifically for men with ED that provides more time for open and frank discussion of treatment and the options available for men with ED and their partners. Nurse-led clinics are being set up across the country—the nurse's role as health educator is vital—but a doctor and nurse working together in this sensitive area of health can provide the quality and continuity of care necessary for these patients. Typically the ED clinic involves an evening clinic consisting of a 20-min appointment with a urologist and a nurse specializing in ED at a hospital. Hormone blood screening for testosterone, prolactin levels and prostate-specific antigen (raised antigen levels would indicate prostate disease) are arranged if appropriate.

7. Financial considerations for Well Man clinic
A detailed calculation of the impact of running a Well Man clinic on the practice accounts will include costs that are both obvious and hidden. Individual practices will have to decide at partnership level how the activity will be funded and whether it is cost effective—the costs that should be considered are:

- Staff costs
- Overheads: such as heat, light, photocopying, correspondence, telephone, etc.
- Computer costs

- Medical, e.g. urine dipsticks and pathology costs
- Equipment, e.g. weighing scales, vitalograph, urinary flow meter
- Hidden costs, such as increased prescribing costs driven by case finding, referral costs for investigation and treatment and increased attendance at follow-up clinics

The source of income for running such clinics also needs consideration. Funding possibilities include health promotion fees, sponsorship, commissioning by a Primary Care Team and patient charges (i.e. private clinic).

8. AUDIT—monitor clinical effectiveness

Audit is vital to ensure that the service is meeting the needs of the local male population and to assess whether the goals of the clinic are being achieved. The method of audit needs to be simple to ensure that practice staff find it user-friendly and to encourage them to keep up to date with the records. It also needs to be focused on specific terms of reference.

The first step when considering audit is to agree standards, then review the progress towards them on a regular basis. Finally, the standards should be reviewed once more to see that they are still appropriate. An example of a standard for ED includes:

1 Offer initial assessment of ED to all patients who request advice and help.
2 Ask all patients affected by predisposing chronic illnesses (including diabetes, hypertension and IHD) a screening question about ED.
3 Keep a register of patients identified as currently or previously having ED.
4 Ensure all patients with ED have all investigations, histories, examinations, management plan and written material recorded in their notes (e.g. instructions re. treatment).
5 Ensure that ALL patients are followed up in accordance with agreed practice policy.
6 Ensure that patients' ED prescription records are reviewed at an agreed interval.

9. Promote the clinic—think laterally

The attitude towards Well Man clinics of those men who have experienced them is very positive. Many men proactively request appointments and wives also arrange appointments for their husbands. However, in terms of targeting those who are most likely to benefit from the clinic, there is still an irony hurdle to overcome. The men who are most likely to attend a clinic are usually in reasonably good health, body aware and indulge in health-promoting behaviour anyway. Hence their attendance at a Well Man clinic, which is simply another step in their health routine. It is encouraging that these men attend, but the real targets for a Well Man clinic are the non-attenders or those who rarely, if ever, visit their surgery.

Non-attenders are more likely to be unhealthy men who think they will be admonished about their lifestyle—for example, those who are overweight or obese, or smoke—and may feel wary about being summoned to the clinic and suspicious if picked out. Young men are particularly difficult to reach as they are not concerned about the long-term results of their unhealthy lifestyle. It is important when promoting the clinic or inviting men to attend, that men realize that the clinic is more than advice about unhealthy habits. It should be billed more as an 'MOT'. In much the same way that men have their cars checked once a year, it should be emphasized that their bodies deserve the same respect and opportunity for an overhaul.

10. Where and when will the service be provided?

The location of the service can be an added incentive to encourage men to attend and can be varied and inventive, as essentially the only requirements for the clinic are privacy, a comfortable environment, a couch for examination, and facilities for blood and urine testing.

The practice could consider working with local businesses to promote the service, or base services in a room or stall in youth centres, unemployment centres, cafes and shops, pubs and clubs, football and sports clubs, gyms and other sports facilities, places of worship, etc.—anywhere where it makes it easy for men to seek advice and makes it 'normal' for them to talk about their health.

In terms of timing, past experience has found that evening, weekend or lunchtime clinics have the best response rate, although attendance can still vary depending on external factors and events. One clinic found that attendances dropped noticeably during the football World Cup or when a James Bond film was on TV!

11. Arrange follow-up meetings

Follow-up meetings with the team should revise how the clinic is functioning, and should be seen as part of the learning process. Team members should be encouraged to be innovative, acknowledge mistakes made and lessons learned. In this way, the team's knowledge base will be increased and confidence in managing men's health problems will be increased.

PUTTING THE THEORY INTO PRACTICE

Using the age/sex register for ease, all male patients between the ages of 35 and 65 could be invited for check-up. The clinic could be held fortnightly in the evening or at midday—choose a night when there are fewer social commitments and men can attend after work. Twenty-five to 30 men could be invited to each clinic and asked to bring a urine specimen. The practice secretary sends the appointments, which are printed by the computer, and marks the cards of the age/sex register to show that an invitation has been issued. If a referral is indicated, an appointment with the doctor should be made before the man leaves the health centre. Records of attendances and outcomes should be kept, and also non-attenders noted. As non-attenders may be the men who would most benefit, another appointment should be issued to non-attenders. During the course of normal surgery, doctors can refer patients to the clinic for a general check-up.

The Letchworth Clinic experience

The target age group for the Well Man clinic at the Letchworth practice is 45–60 years—a list of 1000 men in this age group has been generated by the practice computer. The men are invited by post to attend a regular Tuesday clinic held in the middle of the day by two practice nurses and the health visitor. An open access prostate assessment clinic run by the urology specialist nurse is also available.

The postal invitation results in a 60% attendance rate and non-responders are given a second opportunity to attend at a later date. The clinic also advertises on the practice nurses' notice board and in the practice leaflet. Men identified opportunistically during normal consultations are also filtered into the clinic. A clear protocol is used for the agreed procedures and guidelines and this takes one of the nurses on average 30 min to work through (see sample protocol). Each clinic session lasts 3 h.

GPs are available during the clinic to provide advice and any patients who have abnormalities detected or require further investigation are invited to make another appointment with their GP. If no problems are detected, a repeat appointment in 5 years is offered. Every year, information is collated to assess trends in numbers of attenders, problems detected and outcomes. Attenders are asked to complete a questionnaire designed to assess patient satisfaction and to detect changes in behaviour as a result of attendance. Audit and re-audit are taken seriously to try to assess the value of the clinic.

KEY POINTS TO CONSIDER WHEN ESTABLISHING A WELL MAN CLINIC

- Decide who will provide medical care
- Develop effective team work
- Set goals for men's health
- Arrange meeting to discuss practicalities
- Devise a protocol

- Consider including an ED service
- Financial implications
- AUDIT—monitoring clinical effectiveness
- Promoting the clinic
- Plan time and venue of clinic
- Arrange follow-up meetings

REFERENCES

1   Kirby RS, Kirby MG, Farah RN. *Men's Health*. Oxford: Isis Medical Media, 1999.
2   Pritchard P, Pritchard J. *Practical Guide for General Practice*, 2nd edn. Oxford: Oxford Medical Publications, 1994.
3   Hackett GI. Impotence—the most neglected complication of diabetes. *Diabetes Res* 1995; **28**: 75–83.
4   Riley A, Riley E. Behavioural and clinical findings in couples where the man presents with erectile disorder: a retrospective study. *Int J Clin Pract* 2000; **54**: 220–4.

6

CHAPTER 7

Nurses in the Front Line

The role of the practice nurse in primary care is expanding rapidly. Practice nurses now play an integral part in the setting up and running of diabetic, hypertension and Well Man/Woman clinics. This expansion in role can be attributed to the need to increase provision of care to improve access, the availability of doctors, and the skills and expertise of nurses. Recent policy developments in the National Health Service, including NHS walk-in centres, NHS Direct, and nurse-led personal medical services schemes, have all been based on nurses rather than doctors acting as the first point of contact with the health service.

The concept of nurse practitioners providing front-line care in general practice and in emergency departments, particularly in the management of patients with acute illness, is attracting a great deal of interest. Nurse practitioners are defined as nurses who, following further training, often at graduate level, provide the first point of contact for patients, make independent diagnoses and treatment decisions, managing patients autonomously.

But how do patients feel about being seen by a nurse rather than a doctor? One recent review of 34 studies found that patients are more satisfied with the care they receive from a nurse than from their GP, although there were no differences in health outcomes [1].

The review found a number of explanations for this preference. Nurses were perceived as being able to offer longer consultations and carry out more investigations, as well as offer advice on self-care and managing conditions. Understandably, doctors have more demands on their time (such as administration and home visits), as well as having to deal with a wider range of problems and diseases. However, this review should raise the issue of cost effectiveness in terms of current and future roles of primary healthcare team members in the management of erectile dysfunction (ED).

ROLE OF THE NURSE IN ED MANAGEMENT

If nurse practitioners are to play an integral role in ED management, more autonomy must be given to them, in a variety of disease areas. Sexual health is one area in which nurses have a lot of scope to expand their role and take on more responsibility. The Royal College of Nursing (RCN) has developed its own Sexual Health Strategy that will feed directly into the Department of Health Strategy for Sexual Health. The RCN Sexual Health Strategy aims to have a structure that results in systematic responses to current and emerging sexual health trends, maximizing the voice of nursing at all levels and in all arenas.

With regard to the identification and management of ED specifically, the availability of new and effective oral therapies for the treatment of ED has made it possible for this medical condition to be managed within a primary care environment. Therefore, there is no reason why, with education and training, a practice nurse should not be able to identify and manage ED as part of their remit in general practice.

Nurses who work in general practice settings are generally multiskilled and competent practitioners who come into contact with a huge cross-section of patients who frequently present with a variety of combinations of health problems and needs. Often the nurse is the first member of the healthcare team to come into contact with patients, especially those who are at high risk of having or developing ED, for example, through hypertension or diabetes clinics. Proactive identification of ED in these high-risk groups should be viewed as an integral part of the overall management of patients, e.g. asking 'screening' questions as part of a monitoring programme.

Assessment of ED does require considerable clinical knowledge and skills, and so it must be ensured that the nurse feels able and comfortable to assess and advise patients regarding ED. Practice nurses need to understand their professional boundaries and acknowledge their limitations, just as they would do with any other condition. They should also be aware of the local referral agencies in order to instigate appropriate referral where necessary. It is also advisable to have a clear written protocol, setting out the role of doctor and nurse in the assessment and management of ED in day-to-day clinic work.

There are a number of circumstances where it would be appropriate for the practice nurse to discuss sexual activity with a patient. These include:

- Well Man clinics
- New patient checks
- Specific clinics, e.g. diabetes, hypertension
- Providing repeat prescriptions, especially for those drugs known to be associated with ED
- Female consultations, e.g. family planning clinics/smear tests
- HIV/genitourinary clinics
- Mental health services

Nurses can take reassurance from research which has shown that patients may perceive the practice nurse as being a more appropriate person to discuss their sexual health with than their GP [2]. There are a number of reasons why this might be the case.

- The practice nurse may have developed a role that incorporates more health promotion than that of the GP.
- Practice nurses often have longer consultations than GPs.
- The tasks practice nurses carry out may allow more time for communication [3].

Whilst men may be happy to discuss blood pressure and other problems relating to these conditions with their nurse in theory, in practice, discussing ED may still be difficult. Therefore, it is the nurse's responsibility to initiate discussions on ED with their patients, as men cannot be relied upon to discuss erection problems without prompting.

THE IMPORTANCE OF ASKING ABOUT SEXUAL HEALTH

The RCN published a paper in March 2000 entitled *Sexuality and Sexual Health in Nursing Practice* which stated that:

> '...sexuality and sexual health is an appropriate and legitimate area of nursing activity, and nurses have a professional and clinical responsibility to address it'.

Nurses (and doctors) are taught to regard and respect the individual, care for their needs, support them in times of crisis and distress, and look after the whole body and mind. These principles are integral to the whole concept of healthcare. However, if a doctor or nurse chooses to ignore their client's sexual health then he/she is in danger of providing care that is incomplete and in direct opposition to this holistic approach. Practice nurses must be encouraged to use the opportunities available to them to initiate communication involving sexual health.

While there are a number of nurses who are able and willing to broach the complex and difficult area of sexual health, evidence suggests that many nurses do not feel sufficiently confident or possess the necessary skills to support clients in this area [4], and Webb [5] found that nurses are poor communicators when it comes to discussions about sexuality. There are many reasons why this should be so, but essentially education is the key. It has been found that increased knowledge produces more liberal attitudes and increased comfort when dealing with sexuality in nursing situations [6]. Staff education is a prerequisite if practice nurses are to take a sexual health history with confidence and competence. Sadly, as for doctors, ED does not usually form part

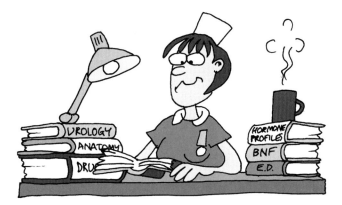

of nurses' basic training, therefore many nurses may feel ill-equipped to raise the subject with their patients. This reticence in discussing sexuality is present at all levels of nursing and it has been suggested that some of the lack of adequate training may even stem from discomfort on the part of the educators themselves [5]. There is a need for education, not only about sexuality itself, but about the associated skills required in talking about sexual health such as communication, teaching and counselling skills.

EDUCATION, EDUCATION, EDUCATION

In order to meet targets for improving the care of patients with sexual complaints, including ED, it is vital that nurses are given high-quality training opportunities. For this to happen, practice nurses must have the backing of their GPs to attend external training courses to develop their knowledge and skills. Nurses should attend courses on prostate disease, ED, hypertension, diabetes and osteoporosis in men to ensure that they have sufficient detailed background knowledge of the most common male-specific diseases in order to run clinics such as a Well Man clinic effectively. Educational opportunities also exist in the surgery. Most GPs possess much of the necessary knowledge and many of the skills required to provide high-quality care for those with ED. These skills can be imparted to nurses in a number of different ways, including training sessions in the surgery, discussion of cases and provision of relevant literature.

It is very important that nurses feel that they have sufficient background information on the aetiology, identification and management of ED to feel comfortable raising the topic with their patients. A fully accredited RCN educational training programme in ED is available, and has significantly contributed to expanding the role of the nurse in the management of ED.

NURSE EDUCATION IN ED

Nurse Education in Erectile Dysfunction (NEED) is an RCN-accredited nationwide training programme that provides nurses with the information and confidence to manage ED. NEED is endorsed by the Royal College of Nursing, the British Association of Urological Surgeons, the British Association for Sexual and Relationship Therapy and the Impotence Association.

NEED was developed with the Royal College of Nursing, an expert multidisciplinary Faculty and 10 nurse ED specialists. Their aim was to produce and implement an accredited programme specifically tailored to the education requirements of nurses which motivates them to:

- Feel confident and competent in the proactive identification and management of ED patients (and their partners) upon completion of the course.
- Play an active part in training a wider audience of nurse colleagues.

NEED was initiated as a sister programme to Erectile Dysfunction in Primary Care (EDiPC), which focused on general primary care education on ED. A survey of participants involved in EDiPC showed that 63% of GPs felt their nurse would be interested in education on ED.

NEED combines a modular and meetings-based educational approach. Area meetings allow NEED participants to consolidate the information in the modules, prepare them to manage ED patients proactively and to run local training meetings for their colleagues.

- NEED provides a comprehensive overview of the aetiology, treatment and management aspects of ED for the nurse.
- NEED provides guidance and confidence for the nurse on the communication and sensitivity issues surrounding ED, when speaking to the patient and/or the partner.
- NEED encourages the proactive identification and treatment of patients at risk and ability to be able to work with the doctor, where appropriate, to formulate a workable screening and management protocol for patients.

For further information on NEED, please go to the website www.edvascular disease.com.

Acknowledgement: This chapter was written with the collaboration of Carole McCallum, Practice Nurse.

REFERENCES

1   Horrocks S, Anderson E, Salisbury C. Systematic review of whether nurse practitioners working in primary care can provide equivalent care to doctors. *BMJ* 2002; **324**: 819–23.

2   Hoolagan T, Blache G. *The Role of the GP in HIV Prevention: Health Promotion in General Practice Report*. London: Hampstead Health Promotions Department, 1993.
3   Jewitt C. *The HIV Project: Sexual History Taking in General Practice*. London: The HIV Project, 1995.
4   Western A. Challenging assumptions. *Nurs Times* 1993; **89**: 26–9.
5   Webb C. *Sexuality, Nursing and Health*. Chichester: John Wiley and Sons, 1988.
6   Payne T. Sexuality of nurses: correlations of knowledge, attitudes and behaviour. *Nursing Res* 1976; **25**: 286–92.

CHAPTER 8

Case Studies

CASE STUDY 1—MYOCARDIAL INFARCTION PATIENT WITH ED

Mr E is 62 years old and suffered a myocardial infarction (MI) 5 months ago, which was treated with thrombolysis. A subsequent treadmill exercise test showed no ischaemia. He is currently taking simvastatin, ramipril, aspirin and atenolol 50 mg and he has a prn TNT spray.

Mr E has not had intercourse with his wife since his MI. They have had one attempt at intercourse but he could not obtain a full erection and so was unable to achieve full penetration. Since then, Mr E has been unable to achieve an erection at all, and both nocturnal and early morning erections appear to be absent. Although his wife is supportive to the idea that they should re-establish their sexual relationship, she is concerned that intercourse could induce another heart attack. Prior to the heart attack their relationship had been normal and they had intercourse approximately once every 10 days.

Mr E admits to a slow urinary stream and gets up twice a night to void. He is an ex-smoker of 10 years and drinks about 8 units of alcohol a week. Although he shares some of his wife's concerns that intercourse may not be safe for him, he feels very frustrated and depressed about his erectile dysfunction (ED) and would like to receive treatment for it.

Examination findings

Weight assessment:	slightly overweight
Body hair:	normally distributed
Genitalia:	normal
Blood pressure:	142/84
Peripheral pulses:	normal
Cardiovascular system:	normal
Neurological examination:	normal

Investigation results

Urinalysis:	normal
Testosterone:	normal
Thyroid function:	normal
Glucose:	normal
Cholesterol:	4.2 mmol/L
ECG:	signs of an old Q-wave anterior infarction

Management considerations

There are many possible causes for Mr E's ED, both psychogenic and organic. Fear on both his and his wife's part that intercourse could induce another MI can interfere with performance, and after one failure Mr E will probably have lost confidence, making further erections difficult. He reports lower urinary tract symptoms, commonly associated with ED, and he has also mentioned that he feels depressed, although this may be a result of his ED as much as a cause of it. He is also on a variety of medications that could be contributing to his ED, but as they all have prognostic benefit he should not be taken off any of them. Bearing in mind all these factors, it is unlikely that Mr E will experience a return of his erections spontaneously.

Suggested course of action

Mr E should perform the treadmill test detailed in Chapter 5 with his wife in attendance so that she can observe his level of physical activity. Both Mr E and his partner should be reassured that intercourse involves no greater level of activity and therefore does not pose any increased risk. Following discussions with Mr E and his partner regarding treatment options, the most convenient and effective treatment option would usually be prescription of a PDE5 inhibitor. However, Mr E is on a TNT spray, which is contraindicated with concurrent use of a PDE5 inhibitor. As these sprays do not have any prognostic benefit and are for symptomatic relief only, and he has no angina, he should be told to discard the TNT spray (this should be documented in the medical notes) and subsequently prescribed a PDE5 inhibitor. Should angina occur during intercourse, he should be advised to cease the exertion, sit on the side of the bed and then stand to reduce preload.

Alternatively, prescription of apomorphine could be considered, although caution is still advised in prescribing apomorphine concurrently with nitrates.

CASE STUDY 2—HYPERTENSIVE PATIENT WITH ED

Mr A is 66 years old and is a retired sales manager. He has been married to his wife for 20 years. She is 56 years old.

Mr A has hypertension, which has been moderately well controlled with bendrofluazide 2.5 mg daily and atenolol 25 mg daily. He also has Type 2 diabetes, which is moderately well controlled with glicazide 40 mg bd.

During a routine follow-up appointment regarding the management of his hypertension, when his general health was questioned, he mentioned that he was not sure whether anything could be done, but he had been unable to achieve an erection for the past 6 months.

Until a year ago, Mr A and his wife enjoyed a healthy sex life, but he has found it increasingly difficult to gain and maintain an erection. Nocturnal and early morning erections are both absent. His libido is good and he would like to have sex at least once or twice a week. His wife has been very patient and supportive; in fact, it was his wife who had suggested that he mention the problem to the doctor.

He smokes 15 cigarettes a day and drinks approximately 26 units of alcohol each week. He believes his problem is simply due to growing old. He has no history of chest pain.

Examination findings

Weight assessment:	obese
BMI:	28
Body hair:	normally distributed
Genitalia:	normal
Blood pressure:	164/92
Peripheral pulses:	poor volume
CVS examination:	normal
Neurological examination:	normal

Investigation results

Urinalysis:	glucose ++
Microalbuminuria:	positive
Testosterone:	normal
Thyroid function:	normal
Glucose:	10 mmol/L
HbA$_{1c}$:	8.2%
ECG:	normal
Renal function:	normal
Cholesterol:	6.4 mmol/L
HDL:	0.8
Ratio HDL/cholesterol:	8

Management considerations

First, it should be noted that both the hypertension and diabetes are only *moderately* well-controlled. Good control of both of these conditions decreases the risk of ED and increases the chance of successful treatment. Therefore the management of both the hypertension and diabetes should be reviewed to see if they can be more effectively controlled, and risk factors addressed.

It should also be established whether there is a temporal relationship between the onset of ED and commencement of the antihypertensive therapy, as there may be a link between the two. If there does seem to be a link, the physician should consider changing the patient's medication to an angiotensin II antagonist or an α-blocker. If ED does not resolve following this, then the physician should consider prescribing a PDE5 inhibitor, especially as this is likely to re-establish nocturnal erections.

Smoking, drinking and obesity are all risk factors for cardiovascular disease and ED, and all of these lifestyle issues will have to be addressed with the patient at some point in the future. In addition to these risk factors, Mr A's microalbuminuria result is positive and his HDL/cholesterol ratio is also typical of a patient with diabetes, indicating that he is at increased risk of vascular disease. Prescription of a lipid-lowering agent and aspirin, once his blood pressure is controlled, should be considered.

CASE STUDY 3—DIABETIC PATIENT WITH ED

Mr B is 60 years old and has been happily married to his wife for 26 years. He was diagnosed with Type 2 diabetes 6 years ago. He also has hypertension, which is poorly controlled (BP 170/100). He is currently taking bendrofluazide (2.5 mg od), atenolol (100 mg od) and metformin (0.5 g tds). He smokes 15 cigarettes per day and drinks about 20 units of beer each week, but to date has ignored advice on curbing his unhealthy lifestyle.

During his last couple of visits to the surgery he has appeared increasingly agitated and with even greater lack of motivation than usual to manage his diabetes on a daily basis.

When the subject of sexual activity is raised, Mr B becomes very embarrassed, but acknowledges he has been having problems with his erections. He reports that he and his wife had previously always enjoyed a 'healthy sex life'. However, for a while now he has found it increasingly difficult to gain and maintain an erection. In fact, for the last 6 months penetrative sexual intercourse has been impossible, as he is unable to get an erection at all. Nocturnal and morning erections are both absent. Although his wife has been very patient and supportive towards the problem, he senses that she finds it frustrating and blames herself that he no longer finds her attractive. The situation has been getting him down and he feels worried and distracted.

He had not mentioned this before because he believed that his problem was due to getting old, although his libido is as good as it has always been. He is relieved to know that his problem has a physical cause, and that neither he nor his wife are to blame.

Examination findings

Weight assessment:	slightly overweight
Genitalia:	normal size and consistency
Blood pressure:	170/100
Body hair:	normally distributed
Peripheral pulses:	poor
Neurological examination:	normal
Cardiovascular system:	due to multiple risk factors, cardiac risk is deemed intermediate, pending further tests

Investigation results

Urinalysis:	glucose ++
HbA_{1c}:	8%
Thyroid function:	normal
Glucose:	slightly raised
Cholesterol:	7.6 mmol/L

Management considerations

It is likely that Mr B's lack of motivation to manage his diabetes and adopt a healthier lifestyle stems from a low mood associated with his ED. Therefore, it would be hoped that treatment of the ED will give him the incentive he needs to control his diabetes more effectively and address his lifestyle.

Diabetes is likely to be the main contributory cause of the ED, suggested by the gradual onset of the ED and a complete absence of erections. His antihypertensive medication could also be contributing to his ED, and in addition he has several cardiovascular risk factors that may be contributing to the problem and could be modified (diabetes, hypertension, hyperlipidaemia and lifestyle). These risk factors also place Mr B in the 'intermediate' cardiac risk group.

Suggested course of action

As Mr B is in the 'intermediate' cardiac risk group, it is very important that his cardiovascular risk is evaluated using the Joint Guidelines CHD risk calculator.

There are major opportunities to reduce risk in this man. Mr B should be encouraged to give up smoking and reduce his alcohol intake. As with case study 2, if a link between his antihypertensive medication and the onset of the ED is suspected, the physician could consider changing the patient's medication. A graduated exercise regime should also be considered and exercise testing would further evaluate risk.

When deciding the best course of ED treatment, it is important to provide patients (and partners) with the full range of treatment options to select from, as this is most likely to improve long-term compliance and satisfaction. A PDE5 inhibitor has an excellent efficacy record in those with diabetes and is the most usual first line approach.

CASE STUDY 4—ANGINA PATIENT WITH ED

Mr D is 50 years old and works in a factory. He has been married for 31 years and has two children. He has hypertension and well-controlled angina. He has been taking atenolol isosorbide mononitrate and aspirin regularly for about 8 years. They were prescribed for his stable angina.

For the past 3 years Mr D has found it increasingly difficult to obtain and maintain an erection sufficient for intercourse, although he does occasionally have nocturnal and early morning erections. In the past 12 months he has managed to have intercourse only once. Although his wife, who is aged 52, has never been particularly enthusiastic about sex, even when they were first married, he reports that she now seems to have completely lost interest in sex. She simply refuses him. He believes that this is because he is not as vigorous as he once was and that she is disappointed with his failures. He loves his wife very much and is keen to resume sexual activity, but sees her lack of interest as his fault. He has a good libido and feels very frustrated about his ED, which he believes must be due to a physical cause. He has been prescribed apomorphine, which, after eight attempts, has still not helped.

Mr D smokes 20 cigarettes a day and drinks 6 units of alcohol per week. He has not told his wife that he is seeking help.

Examination findings

Weight assessment:	slightly obese
Body hair:	normally distributed
Genitalia:	normal
Blood pressure:	146/96
Peripheral pulses:	normal
Cardiovascular system:	normal
Neurological examination:	normal

Investigation results

Urinalysis:	negative
Testosterone:	normal
Thyroid function:	normal
Glucose:	normal
Lipids:	normal
Treadmill exercise test 2 years ago:	no ischaemia

Management considerations

Despite the presence of risk factors for an organic cause for his ED (hypertension, smoking), the fact that Mr D still has occasional nocturnal and early morning erections would suggest that there may be a large psychogenic element to the cause of his ED. His relationship with his wife certainly requires closer scrutiny, as this could be the main reason for his decreasing erectile function. Although he loves her and would appear still to find her attractive, her lack of interest in sex would indicate that she has sexual problems of her own. Even if Mr D's ED is successfully resolved with treatment, his wife will still not be interested in sex, therefore her issues need addressing before therapy is considered for his ED.

Suggested course of action

As Mr D has not yet told his wife that he is seeking help for his ED, the first step is for Mr D to talk to his wife about their problem and encourage her to attend the surgery. Then, provided that they are both in agreement, they should be referred in the first instance to a RELATE counsellor or sexual therapist so that they can discuss their relationship and the reason for his wife's lack of interest in sex.

Following counselling, ED therapy can be considered. A PDE5 inhibitor would be the treatment of choice, but this is contraindicated with Mr D's medication (he is on nitrates). As nitrates have no prognostic benefit for angina, the recommended course of action would be to increase the dose of atenolol to control his hypertension but remove the nitrate. Mr D can then be prescribed a PDE5 inhibitor. As smoking is also a risk factor, it should be strongly suggested that Mr D also addresses his smoking habit. Referral to a stop smoking clinic, or the use of nicotine replacement therapy might be helpful.

CHAPTER 9

Most Frequently Asked Questions

1. HOW SHOULD PATIENT TUITION IN THEIR ERECTILE DYSFUNCTION THERAPY BE MANAGED?

All therapies necessitate adequate training for patients in their use. The GP can either provide this personally or train nurses in the practice. Whoever undertakes the tuition of the patient must take into account the ability and aptitude of the patient on an individual basis, rather than standardized procedure. In most circumstances, provided the patient is in agreement, it is advisable to involve the partner in the training, as their support will be vital to ensure that the therapy is successful. Written material may be helpful, along with information on who to contact in the practice if further support is needed.

2. HOW CAN PRESCRIBING ISSUES BE MANAGED?

As discussed in Chapter 2, erectile dysfunction (ED) treatments are only available on the NHS for a select group of men suffering from specific conditions. Cardiovascular disease (CVD), one of the main causes of ED, is not one of these conditions. If the GP deems a man to be in 'severe distress', the patient can be referred to a hospital specialist for NHS treatment.

The primary healthcare professional must exercise caution and tact when explaining this situation to the patient, as the patient may ask the not unreasonable question: why are men with diabetes more eligible to receive NHS treatment than men with CVD? Cost may well be an issue for many patients, as it is well-known that the incidence of ED is correlated with socio-economic status [1]. There is also a clear link between social class and CVD, one of the main causes of ED, with a significantly higher incidence among men in lower income groups [2]. Men with low incomes who fall outside the framework are least likely to be able to afford a private prescription.

The frequency of repeat prescriptions or the number of doses to be provided per prescription also needs to be addressed. Treatment should be provided on the basis of need, established by the couple's desired frequency of sexual intercourse, taking into account variation between couples. Asking the patient

9

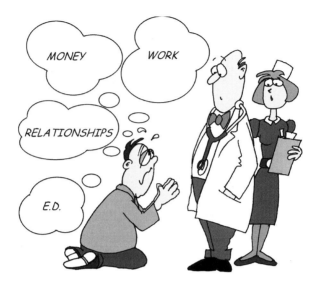

and his partner about anticipated frequency provides the best guide. It is common for there to be an initially high level of enthusiasm (given that the period of abstinence before the patient presented for treatment may well be lengthy), therefore 'rationing' treatment at this initial stage is unhelpful. Most couples settle into a regular and infrequent pattern of sexual activity once this 'honeymoon period' is over. The average frequency of sex amongst adults is around once per week [3]. Estimating usage can be based on the frequency of repeat prescription requests.

Also, the proactive identification and treatment of ED should lead to benefits such as the earlier diagnosis and treatment of risk factors and other conditions such as CVD linked to ED. The benefits of this more effective management should help to offset any additional cost of prescribing through improved treatment outcomes of these underlying conditions. As with any other treatment, the PHCT should not restrict the availability of a drug that can be provided on the NHS.

3. WHAT CRITERIA SHOULD BE USED FOR SECONDARY CARE OR OTHER AGENCY REFERRALS?

Inevitably there will be situations where the assistance of a specialist may be helpful. Situations where a referral would be appropriate include:

- Complex psychological or relationship issues.
- Complex medical problems that may be contributing to their ED, e.g. endocrine or neurological disease.

- Failure to respond to the range of treatments offered at the practice.
- History of complications associated with ED treatments, such as priapism or penile fibrosis.
- Problems involving ethical or other issues the PHCT feels unable to deal with.

4. CAN SILDENAFIL BE TAKEN WITH ANTIHYPERTENSIVES?

Sildenafil is not contraindicated with any cardiovascular medications other than nitrates. It may be thought that as both sildenafil and antihypertensive medications cause a drop in blood pressure, there is a possible risk involved in administering these two treatments concurrently. Although men taking sildenafil while on antihypertensive medication do experience modest effects on their blood pressure (mean change from baseline in sitting SBP/DBP was –3.6/–1.9 mmHg), it has been found that blood pressure returns to pretreatment levels within about 4–6 h [4]. Also, as most hypertensive medications cause vasodilation through mechanisms other than the cGMP pathway, the combination of sildenafil and antihypertensive medications would not be expected to cause synergistic decreases in blood pressure. There has been no incidence of blood pressure-related adverse events in patients taking sildenafil and various antihypertensive medications compared with those taking sildenafil alone [5]. Therefore, acute short-term effects of sildenafil on blood pressure in men with ED is not clinically significant in those taking concomitant antihypertensive medication.

5. HOW SOON CAN SILDENAFIL BE TAKEN ONCE A PATIENT HAS STOPPED TAKING THEIR NITRATES?

There are currently no data on how soon sildenafil can be prescribed after a nitrate has been used or when a nitrate can be taken after sildenafil. The American College of Cardiology (ACC)/American Heart Association (AHA) Expert Consensus Document states that the administration of a nitrate can be considered 24 h after a sildenafil dose, if the patient's haemodynamic response is monitored carefully [6]. It also suggests that sildenafil can be prescribed 1 week after permanent discontinuation of a long-acting oral nitrate, as long as the patient's cardiovascular status has not deteriorated over this time.

For complete peace of mind and to avoid the risk of patients accidentally co-administering sildenafil with nitrates, patients taking sildenafil should be advised not to keep nitrates in the house, and this advice should be documented in the patient's medical notes. Patients taking sildenafil should be advised that if they do experience chest pain during sexual activity, they should cease activity and either sit or stand. This reduces preload and can ease symptoms in a similar way to nitrates. If the angina does not resolve with rest, patients should seek medical advice immediately. Otherwise, patients should routinely consult their family doctor regarding their angina before re-attempting intercourse at another date. If patients accidentally take nitrates concurrently with sildenafil, they should also seek medical attention immediately to have their blood pressure measured. If their hypotension is significant, hospital admission may be required.

6. ARE THERE ANY ADDED BENEFITS FOR PATIENTS TAKING PHOSPHODIESTERASE (PDE5) INHIBITORS BEYOND TREATING THEIR ED?

Preliminary studies suggest that the benefits of PDE5 inhibitor treatment may extend further than just ED. PDE5 inhibitors act by augmenting the actions of nitric oxide (NO) on smooth muscle cell relaxation in the corpus cavernosum, the same process that helps to regulate the basal and stimulated coronary artery tone. This would suggest that PDE5 inhibitors might have a beneficial effect on the smooth muscle of the coronary arteries as well as the penile arteries. This obviously has very positive implications for patients both with CVD and requiring treatment for ED. Currently, most of the studies looking into alternative benefits of PDE5 inhibitors focus on sildenafil citrate.

It should be noted that although the following information outlines potential added benefits of ED treatment, there is currently no licence for sildenafil to be used in these indications and the author cannot recommend the use of sildenafil for these indications.

Improved endothelial function
Acute and chronic low-dose sildenafil treatment in Type 2 diabetic patients has a favourable effect on endothelial function in the brachial artery, therefore potentially helping to prevent cardiovascular events in people with Type 2 diabetes [7].

Pulmonary vasodilation
It has also been found that sildenafil is a potent pulmonary vasodilator which may be an additional treatment option in the management of pulmonary hypertension [8].

Acts as a coronary artery vasodilator
In men with coronary artery disease with stable angina, following administration of 100 mg sildenafil, the time to onset of exercise-limiting angina, total exercise time and also time to 1 mm ST segment depression were significantly increased. Therefore, in men with exercise-limiting angina, sildenafil may potentially facilitate sexual intercourse and general exercise tolerance as well as treat ED [9].

Nocturnal erections and prevention of ED

PDEs may help to prevent ED developing. Sildenafil taken at bedtime produces significantly improved nocturnal erectile activity [10]. As night-time erections contribute to the maintenance of the morphodynamic integrity of smooth muscle cells within the corpora cavernosa, increasing nocturnal erectile activity could help to prevent the deterioration of the cavernosal smooth muscle associated with the ageing process and other vascular risk factors, thereby helping to maintain erectile function.

7. WHEN DECIDING WHICH TREATMENT TO PRESCRIBE FROM THE EVER-INCREASING RANGE OF ORAL THERAPIES, ARE SPEED AND DURATION OF ACTION IMPORTANT CONSIDERATIONS?

Speed and duration of action vary between the different oral therapies. Although upon first glance it might be thought that a fast onset and long duration of action would be desirable in an ED therapy, in practice it would appear that for the majority of men these two factors may not necessarily be the distinguishing vital ingredients of a successful ED treatment. A study into the sexual habits of men with and without ED aged between 40 and 75 [11] found that the average length of time between first deciding to have sexual intercourse to the beginning of sexual intercourse was 53.3 min for those without ED, and 54.2 min for those with ED. Therefore, a therapy providing an onset of action of < 55 min may not be of added benefit when the average length of time required by most men to go from thought to deed is taken into consideration. For the partner, a slightly longer time to onset of action may also be important, as this allows greater opportunity for foreplay.

In terms of frequency of sexual intercourse, current research shows that most men, regardless of whether they have ED or not, have sex just once in 24 h—78% of non-ED sufferers and 87% of ED sufferers reportedly have sex only once in 24 h. This suggests that duration of action may also not necessarily be a deciding factor when selecting the most appropriate treatment for the patient. However, as with any patient, treatment decisions must be a joint, evidence-based decision between the doctor and patient, taking into account the patient's and partner's personal requirements and preferences.

9

8. WHEN MANAGING ED, HOW SHOULD URGENT OR OUT-OF-HOURS PROBLEMS BE ADDRESSED?

Urgent problems arising from use of ED therapy are rare and should not be seen as a major health risk for most patients or as a potential workload problem for the PHCT. As with any treatment, patients should be warned about possible adverse events and how/when they should be managed to avoid medico-legal consequences. For example, patients at risk of priapism (this is mostly a risk for patients using intracavernosal injections) should be given a written protocol providing a full explanation of what priapism is and detailing exactly what they should do if it occurs. There should also be a protocol at the surgery for health staff.

REFERENCES

1 Feldman HA, Goldstein I, Hatzichristou DG, Krane RJ, McKinlay JB. Impotence and its medical and psychosocial correlates: results of the Massachusetts Male Aging Study. *J Urol* 1994; **151**: 54–61.
2 *Office for National Statistics Data*, UK, 1998.
3 Johnson AM, Mercer CH, Erens B *et al.* Sexual behaviour in Britain: partnerships, practices, and HIV risk behaviours. *Lancet* 2001; **358**: 1835–42.
4 Zusman RM, Morales A, Glasser DB, Osterloh IH. Overall cardiovascular profile of sildenafil citrate. *Am J Cardiol* 1999; **83**: 35c–45c.
5 Zusman RM, Prisant LM, Brown MJ, Sildenafil Study Group. Effect of sildenafil citrate on blood pressure and heart rate in men with erectile dysfunction taking concomitant antihypertensive medication. *J Hypertens* 2000; **18**: 1865–9.
6 Cheitlin MD, Hutter AM Jr, Brindis RG *et al.* ACC/AHA Expert consensus document. Use of sildenafil (Viagra) in patients with cardiovascular disease. *J Am Coll Cardiol* 1999; **33**: 273–82.
7 DeSouza C, Parulkar A, Lumpkin D, Akers D, Fonseca V. Acute and chronic effects of low dose sildenafil on endothelial function in type 2 diabetes. 61st Scientific Sessions of the American Diabetes Association. *Diabetes* 2001; **50** (Suppl. 2): A110.
8 Schulze-Neick I, Li J, Petros A, Redington AN. Intravenous sildenafil (Viagra®) and pulmonary vascular resistance in children with congenital heart disease [abstract, P503]. 23rd congress of the European Society of Cardiology. *Eur Heart J* 2001; **22**: 76.
9 Fox KM, Thadani U, Ma PTS *et al.* Time to onset of limiting angina during treadmill exercise in men with erectile dysfunction and stable chronic angina: effect of sildenafil citrate. *Circulation* 2001; **104**: II601–2.
10 Montorsi F, Maga T, Strambi LF *et al.* Sildenafil taken at bedtime significantly increases nocturnal erections: results of a placebo-controlled study. *Urology* 2000; **56**: 906–11.
11 UK study of sexual habits in UK males and their female partners. Prepared for Pfizer by Millward Brown, July 2002.

9

Index

Note: page numbers in *italics* refer to
figures, those in **bold** refer to tables.

accidental death 25
accidents 92
ADAM questionnaire 69
(cyclic) adenosine monophosphate
    (cAMP) 14
adenylate cyclase 14
age, increasing 44
    sexual interest 49
Alma-Ata declaration (WHO/UNICEF
    1978) 26
alprostadil 14
    intraurethral delivery 16, 80
amyl nitrate 10
angina
    case study 113–14
    management 117–18
    mild stable 76
    moderate stable 77
    unstable refractory 78
angiotensin converting enzyme (ACE)
    inhibitors 95
angiotensin II inhibitors 46
antidepressants 45
    sexual dysfunction induction 42
antihypertensive drugs 39, 44, 45, 75
    with sildenafil 117
anxiety 50, 67
    history taking 69
    see also performance anxiety
aortic stenosis 79
apomorphine 11–13
    administration 11
    contraindications 12–13
    efficacy in diabetic patients 81
    mode of action 11, *12*
    nitrate taking 81
    response rates 13
    side-effects 12–13
arrhythmias, high-risk 78
arterial revascularization surgery 21
arteriolar dilatation 4, 5
aspirin 95
atherosclerosis 35, 46
    diabetes mellitus 41
    endothelial cell dysfunction 36
    erectile dysfunction 36, *38*
    non-cardiac sequelae 77
audiovisual stimuli 3
autonomic nervous system 3

β-blockers 46, 65

sildenafil use 81
blood pressure
    reduction 65
    during sex 64
body language 52, 55
body mass index (BMI) 33, 93
Buck's fascia 2
bulbar artery 2

calcium channel blockers 81
cancer mortality **25**, 26
cardiac bypass surgery 40
cardiac valve disease 79
cardiomyopathy, hypertrophic
    obstructive 78
cardiovascular disease
    depression and erectile dysfunction 42
    diabetes risk 33
    early identification of risk 36
    endothelial cell dysfunction 36
    erectile dysfunction 35–6, 37, 38–40
    exercise testing 73
    follow-up of patients 82
    high risk **74**, 78–9
    identification of erectile dysfunction 67–
        9, **70–1**, 72
    intermediate risk **74**, 77
    low risk **74**, 75–7
    management of erectile dysfunction 67–
        9, **70–1**, 72
    management recommendations **74**
    marker function of erectile dysfunction
        28, 36, 54, 116
    mortality **25**, 26
    obesity risk 33
    pathophysiology of erectile dysfunction
        36, 38–40
    patient profiles 75–9
    presentation of erectile dysfunction 34
    risk factors 32–3, 35, 73
    treatments for erectile dysfunction 79–
        80
cardiovascular risk
    assessment 79–80
    potential level 73, **74**
    risk analysis for patient 72–3
    sexual activity 65
cauda equina 43
Caverject *see* alprostadil
cavernosal arteries 2, 5
central nervous system 3, 45
cholesterol-lowering drugs 45
coagulopathies 15
coiled helinous artery 5

coital death 64
colostomy 44
confidence 42
coronary arteries 118
coronary artery bypass graft (CABG) 76
coronary artery disease 35, 36
coronary heart disease (CHD)
    diabetes risk 33
    diabetic patients 67
    early identification of risk 36
    mortality **25**, 26
    national service framework 28
    risk factors 32
    sildenafil efficacy **9**
coronary risk factor identification 28
corpora cavernosa 2, 3
    blood flow in atherosclerosis 41
    nitric oxide signalling mechanisms 41
    smooth muscle fibrosis 15
    smooth muscle relaxation 41
corpus spongiosum 2
counselling
    primary care 60–2
    psychogenic erectile dysfunction 40
    referral 61

death, causes of in men 24, 25–6
depression 4, 42, 45
    endogenous 42
    history taking 69
    reaction to erectile dysfunction 59
    reactive 42
    Well Man clinic 92
detumescence 5
diabetes mellitus
    atherosclerosis of large arteries 41
    cardiovascular complications 67
    case study 111–13
    discussion of sexual problems 51
    early identification 29
    endothelial cell dysfunction 36
    endothelial function 118
    endothelium-dependent vasodilatation
        impairment 36
    erectile dysfunction 40–2
    erectile dysfunction as risk factor 28–9,
        40–1
    female partner 58
    follow-up of patients 82
    heart disease risk 33
    identification in erectile dysfunction
        patient 41–2
    metabolic control 80–1
    National Service Framework 28–9
    pelvic parasympathetic nerve damage
        43
    sexual intercourse risk 67
    sildenafil efficacy **9**
    undiagnosed 33, 42, 54
doctors 88
    availability 102
dopamine receptors D1 and D2 11–12

dorsal vein, deep 3
    ligation 21
drugs, prescription 115–16
    erectile dysfunction 45–6
    repeat 115
drugs, recreational 10, 45
dyslipidaemia 33, 45
    endothelium-dependent vasodilatation
        impairment 36
dyspareunia 58

education
    nurse needs 105–6
    Well Man clinic team members 95–6
ejaculation 5
    delayed 7
embarrassment 51–2, 54, 55
emotional withdrawal 59
endocrine pathology 7
endothelial function 118
environmental factors 26
erectile dysfunction
    assessment 103–4
    broaching 67
    cardiovascular disease 35–6, 37, 38–40
    cardiovascular disease marker 28, 36,
        54, 116
    diabetes mellitus 28–9
    discussion initiation by nurse 104
    disease progression marker 36
    GP treatment 30
    identification 31, 103
    impact 49–50
    incidence 1–2
    maintaining factors 62
    management 103
    marker for cardiovascular disease 28,
        36, 54, 116
    marker for other conditions 34
    neurogenic causes 42–6
    non-vascular cause 42–6
    organic causes 6–7, 8
    pathophysiology in cardiovascular
        disease 36, 38–40
    pathophysiology in diabetic men 41
    patient tuition in management 115
    physiology 5–7
    precipitating factors 61
    predisposing factors 61
    proactive identification 53–4
    risk factors 34
    underlying cause 34
    vascular endothelium 35–6
    venogenic causes 38
    website 91, 106
    Well Man clinic 94
Erectile Dysfunction in Primary Care
    (EDiPC) programme 106
erectile dysfunction service
    consultation time 96–7
    liaison with secondary care providers 97
    requirements for provision 96

secondary care 97
standards 98
erectile dysfunction treatments 7, 8–21
  cardiovascular patients 79–80
  intracavernosal injection therapy 14–16
  onset of action 119
  oral therapy 8–14, 59, 119
  psychosexual therapy 7
  surgical 19–21
  testosterone therapy 21
  transurethral drug application 16–17
  urgent problems 119–20
  vacuum constriction devices 17–19
erectile function
  changes with cardiovascular disease/
    diabetes 67
  nocturnal erectile activity 119
erectile response 58–9
erectile stimulation, psychogenic 3
erectile tissue, arterial flow impairment 7
erection
  inability to maintain 1
  mechanism 3, 4–5
  psychogenic 4
  reflexogenic 4
  self-stimulated 6
  types 4
erection, early morning 4, 6
  loss 7
erection, nocturnal 4, 6
  increasing age 44
  loss 7
  sildenafil 119
exercise
  history 92
  sexual intercourse 64–5, 66
  stroke risk 82
exercise testing 73

fitness 81–2
  aerobic 82

general practitioners
  availability in Well Man clinic 100
  nurse education 105
  see also primary care
glans penis 2
glycaemic control 42
government initiatives for men's health
    26–31
(cyclic) guanosine monophosphate
    (cGMP) 5, 8
  activation 41

health checks, general 31
health education 26
  sexual activity 60
Health of the Nation 26–7
  improvement targets 27
health promotion, effective 26
health risk factors, control 26
health visitor 87

healthcare
  embarrassment 52, 54, 55
  national standards for provision 27–8
  targets 27
  see also men/men's health; sexual health
healthcare professionals
  education 31
  initiation of discussions about sex 53
  language use 56
  sensitive issue discussions 54–6
  see also general practitioners; nurse(s)
heart disease
  death rate reduction 28
  ischaemic 36, 46
  Well Man clinic 94–5
heart failure, congestive 76, 77, 78
heart rate
  reduction 65
  during sex 64, 65
HIV infection 30
homosexual relationships 58
hypercholesterolaemia 36
hypertension 33, 35, 45, 46
  case study 109–11
  controlled 75
  diabetic patients 67
  discussion of sexual problems 51
  endothelium-dependent vasodilatation
    impairment 36
  erectile dysfunction 39
  medication 39
  sildenafil efficacy 9
  uncontrolled 78
  vascular endothelium abnormalities
    35–6
hypogonadism 21
hypothalamus
  dopamine receptors D1 and D2 11
  median preoptic area 3
hysterectomy 59

ileostomy 44
impotence 1, 56
infant mortality 24
insulin resistance 33
International Index of Erectile Function
    (IIEF) 69
interpersonal factors 59, 69
intimacy
  difficulty 7
  needs of female partner 58
intracavernosal injection therapy 14–16
  administration 14–15
  contraindications/side-effects 15
intrapersonal factors 59
Investigation of Limitation of Infarct
    Size 80
irritability 59
ischaemic episodes 73

language use 56
left ventricular dysfunction 77

Letchworth Clinic 100
leukaemia 15
libido
  loss 21, 44
  reduction 69
  see also sexual interest
lifestyle 26
lumbosacral cord ischaemia 43

male-friendly services 86
Massachusetts Male Ageing Study 35
medical assessment 69
men/men's health
  gender gap 24–5
  health goals 90
  inability to discuss health issues 86
  reluctance to seek medical advice 85–6
  taking care of 24–5
  see also Well Man clinic
menopause 59
metabolic equivalent of the task 65, 66, 73
microangiopathy, diabetic erectile
  dysfunction 41
mitral valvular disease 76
multiple sclerosis 43
  sildenafil efficacy 9
multisystem atrophy 43
MUSE (Medicated Urethral System for
  Erection) see transurethral drug
  application
myocardial infarction
  case study 108–9
  emotional drain/stress 67
  history 77
  history and erectile dysfunction 39, 40
  post 76
  recent 78
  sexual intercourse risk 66–7, 81

National Service Frameworks 27–9
  diabetes 28–9
  targets 87
National Strategy for Sexual Health and
  HIV 29–30
neuronal system disruption 7
nicorandil 11
nitrates
  accidental taking with sildenafil 118
  apomorphine use 80, 81
  inhaled 10
  sildenafil contraindication 10–11, 80,
    81, 117–18
nitric oxide 5
  donors 11
  endothelium-dependent vasodilatation
    36
  signalling mechanisms in corpora
    cavernosa 41
  smooth muscle cell relaxation 118
nitric oxide synthase 41
nitric oxide-cyclic guanosine
  monophosphate pathway 5, 10

activation 8
blood pressure regulation 39
nurse(s)
  discussion initiation 104
  education needs 105–6
  general practice 103–4
  role in erectile dysfunction
    management 102–4
  roles 102–6
  sexuality discussion 104–5
  see also practice nurse
Nurse Education in Erectile Dysfunction
  (NEED) programme 105–6
nurse-led services 102
nurse practitioners 102
nurse-run clinics 31
  erectile dysfunction 42, 97

obesity 33
orgasm 5
orgasmic dysfunction 58
osteoporosis risk 93
Our Healthier Nation (1999) 27, 28
outreach clinics 86

parasympathetic nervous system 5, 46
  damage/disease 43
  neural pathways 4
partners
  involvement 59–60
  precipitating factors for erectile
    dysfunction 61
  pregnant 17
  relationship issues 57–9
patient reassurance 67
pelvic region nerve damage 43
pelvic surgery, radical 43
penile artery 2
  atherosclerosis 36
  disease 36, 37
penile prostheses 20–1
penis
  anatomy 2–3
  blood supply 2–3
  defective blood flow 7
  engorgement with blood 5
  flaccid state 4–5
  nerve supply 3
  pain 15, 16
  sensitivity 44
  structural abnormalities 44–5
  structural changes with age 44
  vascular endothelium 35
percutaneous coronary intervention 76
performance anxiety 6, 69
  increasing age 44
  psychosexual therapy 7
peri-prostatic venous complex 3
perineal muscle contraction 5
peripheral nervous system 3, 43
peripheral vascular disease 35
Peyronie's disease 44–5

phosphodiesterase (PDE) type 5 5, *10*
  inhibition 8
  selective inhibitor 8, 13–14, 118–19
physical assessment 69, *71, 72*
poppers 10
practice nurse 87, 103–4
  sexual health history taking 104
pregnant partners, transurethral drug
  application contraindication 17
prematurity 24
prescribing 45–6, 115–16
priapism 119–20
  risk with intracavernosal injection
    therapy 15
primary care 26, 27
  counselling 60–2
  identification of erectile dysfunction 28
  male-friendly services 86
  treatment of erectile dysfunction 30
prostaglandin E$_1$ 14
  intraurethral delivery 16
prostate cancer 43
prostate health 92
prostatectomy, radical
  erectile dysfunction incidence 43
  sildenafil efficacy **9**
psychogenic causes of erectile dysfunction
    6
  cardiovascular disease 39–40
  counselling 60
psychogenic pathways 4
psychological history 69
psychosexual therapy 7, 60–1
  referral 61
psychotherapy 60
pulmonary vasodilatation 118
purpose, sense of 25

quality of life 50, **51**
  maintenance 26
questioning 56–7, 68–9
questionnaires 68–9
questions, open 57

rapid eye movement (REM) sleep 4
receptionists 88
referral 116–17
reflexogenic pathways 4
RELATE 97
relationship issues
  addressing 57–9
  healing 60–2
relationship problems 50, **51**
  psychosexual therapy 7
relationship with partner 49
renal dialysis 44
renal failure 44
  diabetes mellitus in 44

sacral spinal cord nerves 3
Schedule 11 30, 53
secondary care, referral 116–17

selective serotonin reuptake inhibitors
    (SSRIs) 7
self-esteem 25, 42
  loss 50
  woman's 58–9
sensitive issue discussions
  body language 55
  environment 54–5
  terminology 56
  time 55
sex, importance of 49
sex drive 67
sex therapy 58, 60
sexual activity
  cardiovascular risk 65, 79
  discussions with practice nurse
    103–4
  education 60
  fear of resuming/initiating 64
  information on 60
  myocardial infarction risk 81
sexual arousal, woman's role 59
sexual aspiration—achievement gap 49
sexual disorders, female partners 58–9
sexual dysfunction development 64
sexual fantasy 3
sexual frustration, myocardial infarction
    67
sexual health 92
  discussion with practice nurse 103–4
  importance of asking about 104
  strategy 29–31
Sexual Health Inventory for Men (SHIM)
    69, **70–1**
Sexual Health Strategy (RCN) 103
sexual history taking 56–7, 67–8
  interview points 68
sexual intercourse
  as exercise 64–5, 66
  frequency 119
  metabolic equivalent of the task **66**
  myocardial infarction risk 66–7, 81
  myth of danger 64
  patient unwillingness to discuss 51–2
  risks 66–7
  stroke risk 66, 82
sexual interest
  impaired 58
  increasing age 49
  see also libido
sexual performance, lack 7
sexual relationships
  female partner in discussions 58
  vacuum constriction devices 19
sexual satisfaction, decrease 49
sexually transmitted infections 30
sickle-cell disease 15
sildenafil 8–11
  accidental taking with nitrates 118
  administration 8–10
  adverse event risk 80
  antihypertensive medication 117

sildenafil (*continued*)
  contraindications 10–11
  coronary artery vasodilatation 118
  diabetes mellitus endothelial function
    effects 118
  efficacy **9**
  mode of action 8
  nitrate contraindication 10–11, 80, 81,
    117–18
  nocturnal erections 119
  pulmonary vasodilatation 118
  response rates 11
  side-effects 10–11
  use in diabetic patients 81
smoking 41
smooth muscle relaxation 8
social withdrawal 59
spinal cord tumours 43
spinal injury 43
  apomorphine use 13
  sildenafil efficacy **9**
sports, dangerous contact 24
stress 92
stroke 43
  death rate reduction 28
  mortality **25**, 26
  risk 82
  sexual intercourse risk 66, 82
suicide, male youth 25
surgery visiting times 86
surgical treatment for erectile dysfunction
    19–21
sympathetic nervous system 5
  neural pathways 4

tadalafil 13–14
team leaders 88
terminology 56
testicular cancer 26
testicular health 92
testosterone deficiency
  erectile dysfunction 41
  increasing age 44
testosterone therapy 21
trabecular smooth muscle relaxation
    4, 5
transurethral drug application 16–17
transurethral resection of the prostate *see*
    TURP
tumescence 5
  nocturnal 4
  see also erection
tunica albuginea 2, 3
TURP 43
  sildenafil efficacy **9**

unemployment 25
Uprima™ *see* apomorphine
urethra 2

vacuum constriction devices 17–19
  administration 18
  contraindications 18–19
  efficacy 19
  mode of action 18
  side-effects 18–19
  warfarin effects 80
vaginismus 58
vardenafil 13–14
vascular endothelium 35–6
vascular surgery 21
vasculogenic problems 6, 7
veno-occlusive mechanism for erectile
    function 38
  inefficient 7
  pathological causes of failure 38
venous incompetence, ligation 21
Viagra™ *see* sildenafil

warfarin 80
well-being, sense of 25, 49
Well Man clinic 27, 31, 87
  audit 94, 98
  blood tests 93
  clinical effectiveness 98
  complaints 94
  costs 97–8
  data review 93
  developing 87–101
  education for team members 95–6
  erectile dysfunction 94
  erectile dysfunction service 96–7
  examination 93, 95
  financial considerations 97–8
  follow-up 94, 99
  GP availability 100
  heart disease history patients 94–5
  history taking 91–2, 95
  immunizations 93
  investigations 93, 95
  invitations 100
  leadership 89
  Letchworth Clinic experience 100
  location of service 99
  medical care provision 87–8
  men's health goals 90
  non-attenders 99, 100
  nurse education 105
  practicalities 90
  promotion 98–9
  protocol 91–5
  quality of team work 89
  SWOT analysis 88
  team morale 89
  teamwork 87, 88–9
  timing of clinics 99
women
  ability to discuss health issues 86
  role 59